Advance Praise for *Mindful Relation...*

"I LOVE THIS BOOK! Unmanaged stress is such an important detriment to a great relationship. In this very thorough book Dr Bullock provides all the information necessary to manage stress and lead a calm, loving, and meaningful life with SPECIFIC STEPS that anyone can follow. It's a great recipe. As a research-based therapist, I plan on giving a copy of this book to all of my clients."

John Gottman, PhD
Author of *The Seven Principles For Making Marriage Work*

"Relationships are at the core of what defines our humanity and gives meaning in our lives. Yet for many, successful relationships remain a challenge. Dr Bullock, in her ground breaking book, *Mindful Relationships: Seven Skills for Success*, gives us a guide that synthesizes not only her vast personal experience but incorporates the latest research from neuroscience and psychology. Her profound BREATHE model allows us to incorporate this knowledge to not only enhance our relationships but to fundamentally change our lives for the better."

Dr James R Doty, MD, FACS
Professor of Neurosurgery and Director, The Center for Compassion and Altruism Research and Education, Stanford University School of Medicine
New York Times bestselling author of *Into the Magic Shop: A Neurosurgeon's Quest to Discover the Mysteries of the Brain and the Secrets of the Heart*

"Many of us can sit quietly, eyes closed, focusing mindfully on our breath. It is quite another challenge to bring mindful awareness - the ability to be with another human being without judgment, simply seeing this person as he/she is, appreciating all that he/she brings to the situation - into a relationship and to sustain that over time with honesty, compassion, and care. But we can do it, and this is important work for a just and sustainable 21st Century. Dr Bullock gives us a smart and loving guidebook for this work, including both research and humor to motivate us through the difficult challenges of creating healthy, supportive relationships."

Mirabai Bush
Senior Fellow, Center for Contemplative Mind in Society

"I can hardly endorse this book strongly enough. B Grace Bullock has given us a book packed with wisdom, cutting-edge neuroscience, and with her own very unique combination of gifts as a psychotherapist, scientist, and committed practitioner of the contemplative arts. Most importantly, for me, it is an extremely practical and user friendly guide. There is no more complex challenge to the practice of mindfulness than relationships. As Ram Dass used to say, "If you think you're enlightened, go back and visit your parents." Dr Bullock has given us a **method** for bringing mindfulness into relationship — a method which, as she herself points out, is simple and always accessible. Human beings of every stripe will want this book, and will want to give it to their friends and loved-ones!"

Stephen Cope
Senior Scholar in Residence, Kripalu Center for Yoga and Health
Author of *The Great Work of Your Life: A Guide on the Journey to Your True Calling,* and *Yoga and the Quest for the True Self*
Mindful Relationships: Seven Skills for Success

"This book is a must-have resource for leaders and organizations. Dr Bullock offers a compelling account of the most up-to-date science on stress, its impact on relationships and what to do about it. Her coherent narrative is well balanced between research findings, personal stories and interpretation of the relevance to the reader. And her BREATHE model is practical, applicable in the moment, and highly effective. *Mindful Relationships* is remarkably readable. Even the science had me turning the pages as quickly as I could. I highly recommend it!"

Deborah Reidy
Chair, Society for Organizational Learning, North America and President, Reidy Associates
Leadership Development & Executive Coaching

Mindful Relationships: Seven Skills for Success

"B Grace Bullock's book *Mindful Relationships: Seven Skills for Success* is a powerful and user-friendly discussion of what it really takes to develop healthy relationships in the modern world. Her paradigm-shifting explorations explain the role of stress on the relationships we have with ourselves as well as with the people around us. Dr Bullock's mastery of the integration of practice, philosophy, and psychology is evident here. Her expert voice allows the reader to incorporate techniques immediately into everyday life. This is a must-have book for anyone who wants to experience healthy relationships that support their overall well-being."

Felicia Tomasko, RN, E-RYT-500
Editor-in-Chief of *LA Yoga, Ayurveda and Health* magazine, President of Bliss Network

"B Grace Bullock has done the world a great service in writing this book. Her work brings together all aspects of the true relationship experience: what we think, what we feel, how we act and speak, and most importantly, how our bodies and minds register these in real time. It is a valuable contribution to relational science, and an easy pathway to creating better connections with those around us."

Dinabandhu Sarley
Founding member of the Kripalu Center and Past Chief Executive at the Omega Institute

"Elegantly written, meticulously researched, and astonishingly comprehensive, *Mindful Relationships* is the definitive resource for anyone interested in understanding the origins of relationship troubles and how to heal them. As a scientist and clinician, Dr. Bullock is a passionate educator who can explain the neuroscience of stress and the psychological foundation of love in ways useful to us all. From polyvagal and attachment theory 101, Bullock takes us through her own journey of awakening to the power of breath to effect healing for herself and her clients. *Mindful Relationships* will be an important resource for my own work going forward!"

Amy Weintraub MFA, E-RYT500
Author of *Yoga for Depression and Yoga Skills for Therapists* and founder of the LifeForce Yoga Healing Institute

"There is nothing more important than our relationships with ourselves and each other. Yet, there are few resources to help us negotiate these critical and sometimes complicated waters. We all want supportive and effective relationships and most of us just don't know how to make that happen. This important and timely text provides the scientific context, knowledge, and tools needed for deepening personal insight, and strategies for creating positive, effective relationships. This book is a must-have for those of us who want deeper, more meaningful relationships."

Catherine Cook-Cottone, PhD
Associate Professor, University at Buffalo, Yoga and Mindfulness Researcher
Author of *Mindfulness and Yoga for Self Regulation*

Mindful Relationships is a skillful and engaging account of both the science and the consequences and lived experience of the seven skills leading to better relationships for ourselves and others. From the exuberance of someone committed to supporting thriving and joy to the balanced and clear evidence and exercises, Grace's unique background, wisdom and deep commitment shines through each of the chapters."

Daniel Barbezat, PhD
Executive Director of the Center for Contemplative Mind in Society, Professor, Amherst College
Author of *Contemplative Methods in Higher Education: Methods to Transform Teaching and Learning*

"Comprehensively founded in current research and a wealth of personal and professional experience as a scientist, psychologist, educator, and contemplative practitioner, in this book B Grace Bullock has integrated seven practical, accessible skills in the acronym BREATHE designed to deepen and strengthen our relationships with ourselves and others. But make no mistake: this is much more than a mindfulness-based self-help book. From understanding the breath to uncovering the stories we tell ourselves to increasing prosocial behavior, Dr Bullock seamlessly weaves wisdom and knowledge from the fields of neuroscience, mindfulness, and psychology to create a coherent and truly compelling narrative of human nature and the central importance of authentic connectedness to ourselves and to others. And to her great credit, she does so by skillfully incorporating ideas that exhibit, time and again, a deep understanding for the depth and rigor of these disciplines. Dr Bullock's ability to synthesize a diversity of information clearly and insightfully is a true gift for those who want to be more deeply connected to themselves and others, and for those professionals who work with people striving to improve their lives by bettering their relationships."

Kelly M Birch, ERYT-500, PYT 500
Editor in chief, *Yoga Therapy Today*

Mindful Relationships

Seven Skills for Success

Integrating the science of mind, body and brain

B Grace Bullock PhD
Research scientist, psychologist,
organizational innovator

HANDSPRING
PUBLISHING
Edinburgh

HANDSPRING PUBLISHING LIMITED
The Old Manse, Fountainhall,
Pencaitland, East Lothian
EH34 5EY, Scotland
Tel: +44 1875 341 859
Website: www.handspringpublishing.com

First published 2016 in the United Kingdom by Handspring Publishing

ISBN 979-1-909141-70-4

British Library Cataloguing in Publication Data
A catalogue record for this book is available from the British Library

Library of Congress Cataloguing in Publication Data
A catalog record for this book is available from the Library of Congress

Commissioning Editor Sarena Wolfaard
Copy Editor Kathryn Mason Pak
Design Kirsteen Wright
Index Aptara
Typeset DiTech
Printed Pulsio, Bulgaria

The
Publisher's
policy is to use
paper manufactured
from sustainable forests

Dedication

For Margaret Grace Cooper (1921–1995); a woman who embodied compassion, acceptance and loving kindness, and whose spirit lives on in the pages of this book.

Acknowledgments

Just as this book is about relationships, it is also the product of many. It was kindled by numerous conversations with friends and colleagues, each of whom possess a fervent desire to explain and understand this phenomenon we call life, and who possess the tenacity, integrity, and courage to live it deeply, fully, and with abundant curiosity. It was also built on the foundation laid by dedicated scientists, psychologists, clinicians, and educators whose research, theories, and provocative questions have motivated my personal and professional inquiry for decades.

This book was made possible by the gift of time and space offered by my dear friends, Karyn Aho and Ally House. Their friendship, caring, and encouragement motivated me to persevere in this work. I also extend a deep bow of appreciation to Karyn for her astute comments and important input on an earlier draft of the manuscript. Thank you to Mel Bankoff, Tim Danforth, Lisa Freinkel, Cher Mikkola, Deborah Reidy, Elaine Walters, and Erik Westerholm, whose enthusiasm, and rare combination of wisdom, humor, and willingness to read or contribute to the evolution of this book made its writing an act of love and joy. Further, I am indebted to the clients, students, and friends on social media whose insights, stories, and journeys have enriched my heart and inspired the pages of this book, and to Sarena Wolfaard, and the team at Handspring Publishing for their insight and collaboration throughout this process.

I am also thankful for my wonderful dog, Beau, whose presence at or on my feet, and willingness to walk by my side during the months of giving birth to this book made the path much sweeter. Finally, I am profoundly grateful to two significant men with whom I share continuously evolving and deepening relationships. My son Brian, thank you for the gift of your presence, and the depth of your insight. I hope that the world you inhabit, and the people in it, shower you and each other with love and compassion. To my partner, Tim Hicks, thank you not only for reviewing multiple drafts of this manuscript, and for supporting me and this work without fail, but for bringing new meaning to what it is to be in a healthy, fulfilling, and loving relationship.

Contents

No act of kindness, no matter how small, is ever wasted.

Aesop

Note

The details of the individuals described, including name, age, gender, ethnicity, profession, familial relationship, place of residence, and history, have been changed. Any resemblance to persons living or dead resulting from changes to names or identifying details is entirely coincidental and unintentional.

Introduction

If civilization is to survive, we must cultivate the science of human relationships – the ability of all peoples, of all kinds, to live together, in the same world at peace.

Franklin D. Roosevelt

Relationships are fundamental to our health and happiness. Yet, we may find ourselves engaging in behaviors that weaken our social ties. One of the main reasons why this occurs is that many of us live in a state of chronic stress. When stressed, we inhibit the brain's valuable resources responsible for encoding, processing, retrieving, and responding to, complex information. Our perceptions become distorted, our minds become rigid, and our capacity to listen is greatly reduced. We become inattentive, impatient, and less accepting of others' differences. Stress hampers our ability to respond to others mindfully, and increases the probability that we will behave thoughtlessly and reactively. Consequently, we run the risk of hurting those around us and damaging our relationships.

Life stress refers to any situation that challenges our physical and psychological balance. Although not all stress is unhealthy, circumstances that we perceive to be unanticipated, uncontrollable, or distressing can lead to physiological, emotional, cognitive, and behavioral dysregulation, particularly when they are persistent. Many of us are so accustomed to chronic stress that we are desensitized to it. We assume that relentless pressure is a natural part of life, even if it undermines our social bonds, and harms the systems in which we live and work.

In our quest to get more done in less time, we have become distracted multi-taskers. When juggling too many elements, we listen absent-mindedly, respond halfheartedly, and inadvertently discount others. This lack of attentiveness creates depersonalization and disconnection, and conveys the false impression to others that they are unimportant. The digital era only adds to this phenomenon. Because much of our communication takes place via screens rather than in person, our ability to observe the subtleties of nonverbal cues is virtually eliminated. Technology-based communications allow us to turn each other on or off at will, and to circumvent messages that we consider disagreeable or painful. If we don't like what we hear, we can dismiss or delete a message, "unfriend" the author without their knowledge, or turn off a device without experiencing the relational consequences of our actions.

But we have the power to interrupt this cycle of chronic stress and relationship dysfunction, and to create lives and relationships that reflect the goodness in our hearts rather than the turmoil of our minds. It begins with taking responsibility for our stress level, caring for ourselves, prioritizing our relationships, and using the tools at our disposal to create healthy, satisfying, and fulfilling connections.

Relationships take many forms. They may include spouses or partners, family members, friends, colleagues, teammates, or exist within social, political, and religious contexts. You even have a relationship with yourself. Regardless of the nature of the connection, relationships come with responsibility. We are called upon to listen, attend, and communicate, even when things get difficult. But that doesn't always happen.

In the many years I have worked as a psychologist, researcher, educator, and leader, I have heard many stories of those who were disappointed, disillusioned, or emotionally wounded in relationships. In some cases, it was the result of parents, caregivers, or family members who were dismissive, unsupportive, absent, neglectful, or abusive. In others, intimate relationships and close friendships contained physical or emotional aggression, betrayal, abandonment, or deceit. For many, inhumane working conditions, political oppression, institutionalized racism, economic and social disadvantage, and discrimination have left them injured and mistrustful. Regardless of the context or magnitude of dysfunction, one factor remains constant – people are most often hurt when individuals or systems are highly stressed, inattentive, reactive, nonresponsive, or unwilling to examine the impact of their actions or mindsets. This is why taking responsibility for ourselves, and mitigating the effects of chronic stress, is essential to our health and wellbeing.

This book represents years of formal and informal exploration of why we flourish, why we don't, and what differentiates a positive relationship experience from a negative one. It is the culmination of several decades of research, observation, and conversations with friends, clients, students, and workshop participants, each of whom were generous enough to share their stories. This investigation led me to several important conclusions. First, our social bonds define the quality of our lives. Second, chronic stress often weakens these connections. Third, by breathing intentionally, we can induce parasympathetic nervous system dominance, defuse the stress response, and increase our resiliency to challenging life events. This gives us access to the cognitive and emotional resources necessary to interact with others successfully.

Why the Breath Matters

Breath is life. Nearly every living organism must breathe to survive. Without breath, we expire. In December of 1997, I nearly did. It was almost Christmas. A dim grey light from a distant window and the squeak of shoes on linoleum signaled a new day. I survived another marathon night of tubes, masks, and fluorescent lights. Days before, an infection triggered a fire in my asthmatic airways leaving me gasping for air like a fish out of water. My chest heaved. My neck and shoulder muscles wrenched up and down. Exhaustion permeated every cell of my being. Only one thing mattered. "Breathe," I recited over and over again. "Breathe."

After four days of my hospitalization at the UCLA Medical Center, the attending physician and her circle of medical residents arrived looking grim. Respiratory therapy had failed and they feared it would only be a matter of hours before I wouldn't be able to breathe on my own. She recommended a respirator. I refused. Deep down, I knew that fighting for each breath was all that was keeping me alive. I wasn't about to give that up. Instead of consenting to the respirator, I agreed to aggressive drug therapy that made me violently ill. By some miracle, days later the weight from my chest lifted, and the burning in my lungs eventually began to ease. For the first time, I slept and held down a bit of food. As I drifted in and out of consciousness, I recited my mantra over and over. "Breathe. Breathe. Breathe." I was discharged from the hospital on Christmas Day, vowing never to return.

In the months of recovery that followed, I began to track my breath even more closely. I noticed that when my breathing was shallow or my chest was tight, I felt more agitated, anxious, or fearful. My entire body contracted in on itself in a defensive posture, compressing my lungs and the muscles surrounding them. The more I tensed up, the harder it was to breathe and the more stressed I felt. What's more, I observed that the vicious cycle of shortness of breath, stress, fear, and defensiveness was negatively impacting my relationships. The more uncontrollable my life felt, the less able I was to cope with even mundane interactions effectively. I interpreted others' behavior as irksome, intrusive, or undesirable, and tended to withdraw my attention and affection, or to respond with irritability rather than kindness.

In the years that followed, I began to pay rapt attention to my breathing, slowing it down whenever I could. It was very difficult at first. My body was used to its habitual, defensive pattern of rapid and shallow respiration. When I tried to slow my breathing down, I often felt as though I wasn't getting enough oxygen – and it scared me. But, over time, things shifted. With practice, I was able to let go of the vice grip of fear and my obsessive thoughts that I wasn't getting enough oxygen. Then something remarkable happened. Breathing became easier. I had fewer asthma attacks. The muscular body armor that had defended me against my illness began to soften. I felt more at ease and more able to face the challenges of my life, my work, and my relationships.

This experience was so transformative that it led me to pursue a doctorate in clinical psychology, with an intensive study of neuroscience, behavioral genetics, and psychophysiology. My research initially focused on the link between a parent's thoughts and feelings about his or her child, and how these beliefs played out in parent–child interactions. In 2007, I published a now widely used method for assessing "relational schemas" – a person's thoughts and feelings about a close other. It was here that I discovered how profoundly the stories that we tell ourselves dramatically shape our behavior in relationships, often outside of conscious awareness.

Over time I began to shift the emphasis of my research, teaching, and writing from seeking to understand the interpersonal dynamics that contributed to poor child and adolescent developmental outcomes, to exploring the link between mind, body, brain, and psychological experience. With the breath as my anchor, I delved into the scientific literature to satisfy my curiosity about a number of key questions. How do we breathe? What does science tell us about the relationship between breath, mind, emotion, and behavior? If we alter our breath, can we alter our thoughts, emotions, or experience? Can we change our behavior and our relationship with ourselves and others by intentionally modifying our breath cycle? If so, how? Lastly, what are the larger social implications of bringing this intentionality of breath and mind into the domain of relationship, and the systems in which we live and work?

As all of this was going on, I began practicing yoga and meditation, through which I experienced the remarkable impact of breath modification and the mind–body connection, and the ways in which contemporary clinical psychology had largely overlooked the profound influence of bodily states on cognition, emotion, and behavior. At that time, I had been trained, like most mental health professionals, to consider people from the neck up, having little awareness of the extent to which issues truly are stored in our tissues. As I became increasingly interested in mind–body medicine and research, I turned to the study of biomechanics, motor control, and human physiology, assuming that Western science held the answer to this mystery. But I came up short. I then shifted my focus to an intensive study of Eastern healing traditions that incorporate mindfulness and the breath as key elements in the shaping of experience, and the cultivation and maintenance of good health.

As my ideas regarding the mind–body relationship evolved, so did my work with clients, students, and workshop participants. Inspired by these interactions and experiences, it became clear that it is difficult, if not impossible, to be self-aware, change behavior, and be present and effective in our relationships when in a persistent state of stress. Research in neuroscience and psychophysiology shows that, when we are acutely or chronically stressed, our ability to listen and effectively process information is severely impaired, and our behavioral repertoire is greatly restricted. More importantly, when in states of heightened physiological arousal, capacities like attention, present-focused awareness, empathic understanding, and effective communication, all of which are necessary to be socially and emotionally attuned to others, are attenuated.

The BREATHE model – an approach that integrates the wisdom of contemporary neuroscience, psychophysiology, cognitive and behavioral psychology, stress and emotion research, and the wisdom of Eastern contemplative traditions – is the outcome of this exploration. The model includes seven skills that are organized around the following premises.

1. It is very difficult, if not impossible, to act skillfully, remain focused and aware, and respond to others from a place of clarity and intentionality when we are chronically stressed.

2. Physiological homeostasis, or balance, is necessary to create space for mindful, present-focused awareness of the physical, emotional, and cognitive states that shape our behavior and experience.

3. Breath modification is the most accessible and immediate tool that can be used to attain physiological balance.

4. When in states of homeostasis, we are better equipped to process stress, and to understand the stories that we tell ourselves about our lives and relationships. We are also able to explore the ways in which these narratives can distort our lens of perception. This allows us to remain more grounded in the present moment.

5. When anchored in the present moment, we are more likely to act skillfully, increasing the probability that we will cultivate and experience successful relationships. This capacity to be present is inherently mindful.

The BREATHE model emphasizes decreasing stress, increasing stress resilience, and present-focused awareness as key tools for cultivating self-regulation, self-understanding, and socio-emotional intelligence. Its principles enable you to become both an active observer and a participant in your life. The tools are neither complicated nor remarkable. Most find them easy to learn and practice and many report that the seven skills are empowering and transformative.

In addition to being the product of many years of inquiry, this book was inspired by the many remarkable teachers, students, clients, colleagues, and friends with whom I have explored the workings of the mind, body, and brain and the ways in which dysfunctional thoughts, feelings, and movement patterns can influence our experience. This can include everything from anxiety, panic, obsessive compulsive disorder, and post-traumatic stress disorder to depression, substance use, relationship crises, fear of falling, osteoporosis, respiratory illness, and chronic pain.

During the past several years I have explored this work in the context of decision-making and individual and organizational behavior. Prior to beginning my career as a psychologist and researcher, I spent nearly a decade working in the corporate world, where, as the Director of Business Development for a large architectural firm, I spent a great deal of time working with an exceptional team of leadership consultants hired to assuage the growing pains of a rapidly expanding firm during turbulent times. I developed a keen interest in organizational psychology and systems change. When you consider that most of us spend the overwhelming majority of hours each work day navigating the sometimes difficult terrain of organizational life, it seems more important than ever that we learn to negotiate our relationships successfully. I've observed that the same issues that plague individuals – chronic states of stress and personal stories characterized by mistrust, fear, despair or inadequacy – also impact our professional milieu. Just as the seven skills can enable people to experience agency in their personal lives, they also work in the business realm to cultivate socio-emotional intelligence, mindful awareness and compassionate organizations and systems.

Years ago, when I began my quest to understand the breath and its relationship to experience, I viewed it as a mechanism for survival. I had no idea then that survival would involve not only the mind and body, but our relationships and the systems that we inhabit as well. Once I recognized and began to investigate the connection between the breath and lived experience, and the integral role that physiology plays in our interactions with others, the genie was out of the bottle. I would never see my work in the same way again.

PART 1

FOUNDATION

The main task in life is to give birth
to our self to become what we
actually are.

Erich Fromm

1 | Why Relationships Matter

Life isn't about finding yourself. Life is about creating yourself.
George Bernard Shaw

Relationships are essential. From neurons to neighborhoods, we are webs of interconnectedness. The bonds we form with others nurture and sustain us physically, mentally, and emotionally. We learn about the world by exchanging thoughts, feelings, ideas, and experiences. We rely on community to create, produce, and supply everything from food, shelter, and clothing to education and entertainment. As Austrian-born philosopher Martin Buber noted in his influential book, *I and Thou*, human life finds its meaning in relationship. In the absence of connection, we are less able to live happy, fulfilled lives (Buber 1971).

The very nature of life is one of union. We are created by the coupling of gametes that rapidly proliferate into communities of miraculously organized cells. Gestation is an interdependent process between mother and child. From birth onward, we require touch, sound, and reciprocal interaction to inspire the formation of neural networks and structures essential for learning, memory, emotional processing, self-regulation, and myriad other capacities essential to our biological and socio-emotional flourishing (Harlow 1959; Bowlby 1998). Early relationships are so pivotal to development that children who lack sufficient touch or social engagement fail to thrive (Poland & Ward 1994; Marcovitch 1994; Pearce & Pezzot-Pearce 2007).

Although the brain appears to be a solid mass of folded tissue, it is actually a highly social structure. It is comprised of neurons that function in communities called neural networks. Some of these networks are dedicated to processing, interpreting, and making meaning of relational experience. Others specialize in imitation, attunement with others, emotional resonance, and empathy.

Although the brain is wired to process, interpret, and learn from social input, the extent to which it fulfills its destiny depends on experience, particularly during stages of growth, pruning, disorganization, and reorganization. During such critical periods, children depend on the emotional availability of, and reciprocal interactions with, caregivers to kindle the formation of neural networks dedicated to self-regulation, emotion-regulation, distress tolerance, and resilience. But development does not end there. The size, shape, and architecture of the brain continue to be experience-dependent throughout the lifespan. In other words, brain development, maturation, and change depend a great deal on our relationship to others and the natural world (Bakermans-Krananburg, van Ijzendoorn, & Juffer 2008; Cozolino 2014; Tucker, Luu & Poulson 2006).

Attachment Styles and Relationship Behavior

Like brain development, social bonds exert considerable influence on psychosocial maturation. Attachment theory, first proposed by twentieth century British psychiatrist and psychoanalyst John Bowlby, provides a comprehensive framework for elucidating how interactions with caregivers early in life set the stage for later relationship experience (Bowlby 1998). Inspired by evolutionary biology, ethology, developmental psychology, cognitive science, and systems theory, attachment models suggest that a primary caregiver's responses to the biological, environmental, emotional, and cognitive needs of a child create a set of expectancies for subsequent relationships. Reliable, nurturing, caregiving during childhood is associated with healthy, adaptive psychosocial development. Conversely, unreliable or absent caregiving is linked to a broad range of biopsychosocial problems that can persist into adulthood (Ainsworth 1969; Ainsworth et al. 1978; Bowlby 1998; Lyons-Ruth et al. 2013).

Attachment researchers generally agree that child attachment styles fit into one of three categories: secure, anxious-ambivalent, and avoidant. These categories were designed to describe not only behavioral patterns, but also how individuals develop expectations of others with whom they share relationships (Ainsworth et al. 1978). Numerous observational studies find that securely attached infants and young children rely on caregivers as a secure base while exploring their surroundings, and tend to seek contact with, and are comforted by, their caregiver following a period of separation. Conversely, infants with an anxious-ambivalent style alternate between seeking and resisting contact with their caregivers following separation, and those with an avoidant attachment style neither exhibit distress when separated from a caregiver, nor seek contact upon the caregiver's return. In general, longitudinal research suggests that children who are insecurely attached experience higher rates of depression and anxiety, difficulties in relationships with peers, and deficits in social skills, social identity, and intellectual development (Ainsworth et al. 1978; Berlin, Cassidy, & Appleyard 2008; Berlin, Zeanah, & Lieberman 2008).

Adults have similar attachment styles to those identified in children. Securely attached adults tend to view themselves, others, and their relationships positively, and are able to balance the need for independence with those of intimacy and connectedness. Anxious-preoccupied adults, on the other hand, struggle with intimate relationships, often being highly anxious, ambivalent, insecure, dependent, or requiring a great deal of approval and reassurance. Adults with a dismissive-avoidant pattern harbor negative views of relationships, seeing themselves as fiercely independent, self-sufficient, and not in need of close or intimate relationships. Lastly, fearful-avoidant adults tend to desire more, but seek less intimacy, suppress their emotions, mistrust their partners, and feel very uncomfortable in close relationships (Bartholomew & Horowitz 1991; Berlin, Cassidy, & Appleyard 2008; Hazan & Shaver 1990, 1994).

Approximately 50% of adults have a secure attachment style. The rest can experience even healthy relationships as challenging, and create safety, security, and predictability in dysfunctional ways. Insecure, avoidant, ambivalent, anxious, or dismissive attachment styles can manifest as jealous, insecure, angry, fearful, or excessively dependent behavior, as well as an overwhelming desire for intimacy, struggles with communication, and the refusal or inability to form intimate bonds (Bartholomew & Horowitz 1991; Berlin, Cassidy, & Appleyard 2008).

Whether characterized by a secure or insecure attachment style, one thing is for certain when it comes to relationships: they are often accompanied by powerful emotions. According to Bowlby, "Many of the most intense emotions arise during the formation, the maintenance, the disruption, and the renewal of attachment relationships," (Bowlby 1980, p. 40). "The formation of a bond is described as falling in love, maintaining a bond as loving someone, and losing a partner as grieving over someone. Similarly, threat of loss arouses anxiety and actual loss gives rise to sorrow; whilst each of these situations is likely to arouse anger. The unchallenged maintenance of a bond is experienced as a source of joy" (Bowlby 1980, p. 40).

One way we attempt to navigate the unpredictable emotional terrain of a relationship is by creating internal working models. Often based on our attachment style, these models shape the stories that we tell ourselves about how relationships work and what to expect from others. We use these heuristics to inform the assumptions and expectations we hold about how others perceive us, as well as our rules of conduct (Bullock & Dishion 2007). As we will see in later chapters, these stories can markedly impact our experience, leading us to make choices and engage in actions that can enhance or undermine the quality of our lives.

Relationships and Health

In addition to having considerable influence on trajectories of neurological and social development, the ability to foster and maintain close relationships significantly impacts physical and mental health (Cohen 2004; Feeny & Collins 2015; Haslam et al. 2009; Cobb 1976; see Umberson, Crosnoe, & Reczeck 2010 for a review).

Social connection is one of the strongest predictors of longevity (House, Landis, & Umberson 1988). In 1979, Lisa Berkman, director of the Harvard Center for Population and Development Studies, co-authored an important, nine-year, prospective study of a random sample of nearly 7,000 adults in the Alameda County Study. Results showed that participants who reported fewer social ties like marriage, contact with friends and relatives, and church affiliation at the beginning of the study were more than twice as likely to die during a nine-year follow-up period. This effect was not related to behaviors like drinking, smoking, or a sedentary lifestyle (Berkman & Syme 1979).

In a meta-analysis of 148 studies with over 300,000 individuals examining the relationship between human interaction and health outcomes over an average of seven years, researchers at Brigham Young University found that a relationship of any sort, whether good or bad, improved a person's odds of survival by fifty percent. What's more, the magnitude of these effects was equivalent to quitting smoking, and exceeded many other health risk factors for premature death such as obesity and inactivity (Holt-Lunsad, Smith, & Layton 2010). Theories of social support suggest that relationships may serve to buffer the negative effects of stress including distress- and pain-related neural activity in the brain (Cohen & Willis 1985), which may help to improve overall health outcomes.

In as much as relationships can enhance wellbeing, research shows that the absence of close bonds may be hazardous to your health (Cohen 2004; Hawton 2010; House, Landis, & Umberson 1988). Several review articles offer consistent evidence that a lack of quality social relationships is linked to a host of health conditions including autonomic dysregulation, hypertension, cardiac disease, cancer, slower cancer recovery, and delayed wound healing (Ertel, Glymour & Berkman 2009; Everson-Rose and Lewis 2005; Robles & Kiecolt-Glaser 2003; Uchino 2006). Studies also consistently show that separation from others, or from a spiritual or religious source, presents a significant risk for heart disease, even above and beyond lifestyle risk factors like smoking, obesity, a high-fat diet, and a sedentary lifestyle. For example, one investigation of 655 patients who experienced a stroke revealed that those who were socially isolated were two times more likely to have another stroke within five years compared to those with strong social ties (Boden-Albala et al. 2005).

Poor relationships, low marital satisfaction, marital hostility, and divorce can also negatively impact wellbeing (Eaker et al. 2007; Kiecolt-Glaser 1999). Individuals in unsatisfying marriages tend to experience higher rates of loneliness and depression, and have poorer immune function than happy spouses. Studies show that both newlyweds and older married couples with poorly managed marital conflict have higher levels of stress hormones like epinephrine and norepinephrine, and show evidence of immunosuppression. These effects are greater for women than men. What's more, divorced and separated individuals tend to fare worse physically and mentally than widowed, married, or single adults, often having the highest rates of acute and chronic health problems, in addition to higher death rates from infectious diseases (Gleason et al. 2003; Karney & Bradbury 1995; Wills 1991).

It is important to note that the nature and quality of relationships have significant bearing on their health-enhancing properties, and that this relationship remains a mystery. Studies find that, for some, increased relationship distress may be linked to improved health behaviors (Krause et al. 1993; Lewis & Rook 1999). Others find that even negative relationships may serve as a protective factor. For example, a 19-year longitudinal study of adults found that lower levels of support and increased relationship negativity were associated with higher levels of mortality, but that even negative relationships were better than no relationship at all for those with chronic illnesses (Birditt & Antonucci 2008). Even so, supportive relationships appear to be of greatest benefit to physical and psychological wellbeing (Cohen & Willis 1985; House et al. 1988; Umberson et al. 2010).

Workplace relationships are also closely linked to wellbeing. Supportive work ties are associated with immediate and long-lasting psychological benefits and cardiovascular, immune, and neuroendocrine system health as well as being emotionally energizing. Negative or toxic workplace relationships, on the other hand, deplete psychological resources and decrease wellbeing and vitality (Dutton 2003; Heaphy & Dutton 2008; Quinn 2007). Collectively, the research concurs that social bonds are important for maintaining physical and psychological wellbeing at home and at work. In spite of this knowledge, we aren't always able to engage our relationships as fully or effectively as we would like. For many, this occurs because chronic stress depletes our physical and psychological resources, leaving us less able to adapt to the demands of life or respond the needs of others.

Social Relationships and Stress

In 1956, renowned psychologist Hans Selye introduced the term "stress" to represent anything that threatens homeostasis – the internal state in which our body is in balance and operates efficiently and sustainably (Selye 1956). From that word came "stressor," an actual or perceived threat that triggers the "stress response" – a state of physiological arousal that occurs in response to a real or imagined threat (Lazarus & Folkman 1984).

Our experience of stress is intimately woven into the fabric of our relationships. High levels of chronic stress can threaten social bonds, whereas connection to others can buffer the effects of crisis (Cohen & Willis 1985). This buffering effect can occur across a number of dimensions of physical and psychological health including diminishing neural and physiological reactivity to social stressors (Eisenberger et al. 2007). In a review of the research examining the effects of social support on mitigating stress, Cohen and Willis found that supportive relationships consistently ameliorate the effects of high levels of stress, and that this effect may be the result of increased self-esteem and feelings of personal agency and effectiveness. In other words, receiving support from others may make us feel more capable of tackling life's problems, and feel better about ourselves on the whole (Cohen & Willis 1985).

Marriage and family researchers have long sought to understand the mechanisms that support or detract from healthy relationships. In a review of the research on the longitudinal course of marital quality and stability, psychologists Karney and Bradbury found that marital success is shaped by a number of factors. One of these is appraisal, or how an individual perceives the benefits of a relationship compared to its costs. Karney and Bradbury theorize that a relationship remains intact when satisfaction with the relationship outweighs dissatisfaction, or when the tangible or psychological cost of leaving the relationship is perceived as greater than the unhappiness created by staying put. Dissatisfaction occurs because couples have difficulty managing conflict, or resort to critical, hostile, dismissive, or coercive styles of engagement instead of effective problem solving (Karney & Bradbury 1995). Relationship longevity may also be influenced by attachment styles, how well couples negotiate independence and interdependence, and the extent to which they receive community (Hazan & Shaver 1987, 1990, 1994).

Karney and Bradbury (1995) also explored the link between adaptation to internal and external stressors, and relationship quality and sustainability. They concluded that stress and poor coping strategies feed "… a vicious cycle whereby (a) stressful events challenge a couple's capacity to adapt, (b) which contributes to the perpetuation or worsening of those events, (c) which in turn further challenge and perhaps overwhelm their capacity to adapt." (p. 24). In short, stress and vulnerability to stress can impede a couple's effective coping, which can determine whether or not a marriage inevitably succeeds or fails.

No matter the context or the circumstances, relationships can be challenging. They require us to be vulnerable, and to shed layers of self-protection in order to see and be seen, to love and be loved. Whether intimate partner or adversary, those with whom we share social bonds are often our greatest teachers. In good circumstances or bad, most relationships compel us to face painful realities about our self, and those we are connected to. It is through learning to be with others that we discover what we value, and how we choose to be in the world.

Relationships also compel us to examine how our behaviors affect others. Often the impact of our actions is mirrored back to us in all its grit and glory. When we are content, we convey kindness and are greeted with enthusiasm. When we are tired, angry, chronically stressed, or overwhelmed we communicate frustration, impatience, irritability, and intolerance and are likely to elicit aggression, hurt, and withdrawal.

Many of us live in a state of chronic stress. Part of this stress often stems from the extent to which we are barraged by technology. Many of us are tethered to our phones and devices, compelled by the need to multi-task and stay connected with the world around us. When divided, our capacity to attend to the person or task at hand is reduced, and something inevitably suffers. People notice our lack of engagement. Our performance declines. We become less effective at work or more alienated at home. Feelings get hurt. We feel awful. This causes even greater strain. Eventually we find ourselves caught in a stress cycle.

Many of my clients, students, and workshop participants report experiencing this vicious cycle, and I have certainly felt it in my own life. The demands of work, finances, family, and social responsibility fuel a persistent, almost obsessive drive to accomplish, believing that the more we do, the less vulnerable we will be. Sadly, this strategy doesn't usually work.

The good news is that we have the capacity to change our experience and relationships. It all begins with taking responsibility for our thoughts, feelings, actions, and level of stress, and setting an intention to do things differently. This doesn't necessarily mean that life will change overnight, but with a newfound awareness of how the mind and body support resilience and the role that our thoughts, feelings, and actions play in creating our experience, we can practice new ways of thinking and being and more effectively relate to ourselves and our friends, loved ones, colleagues, and the world at large. As Chinese mystic and philosopher Lao Tzu once said, "The journey of a thousand miles begins with a single step."

2 | Understanding Stress

Life is not a problem to be solved, but a reality to be experienced.

Søren Kierkegaard

Stress generally refers to any ongoing demand without a known ending that threatens or exceeds the physical and/or psychological resources that an individual can mobilize (Lazarus & Folkman 1984; Selye 1956). Each time we encounter a challenging circumstance, the body and brain initiate the stress response. This response heightens sympathetic nervous system (SNS) activation and increases cardiopulmonary, endocrine, immune, musculoskeletal, and nervous system output. This helps to facilitate active coping strategies like jumping out of the path of an oncoming car, or focusing attention on a difficult problem. These physiological reactions are adaptive in the short term, but are harmful when sustained for extended periods of time because they were not designed for persistent, long-term use.

The Two Forms of Stress

Stress can be categorized into two primary forms: eustress, which can be considered a healthy form of stress, and distress, which is generally considered to be unhealthy, particularly when chronic (Selye 1956). Eustress relates to experiences that motivate us to expand beyond our current limits, and inspire us to be creative, resourceful, or break new ground. It is linked to adaptive coping, innovation and achievement. Examples include running a marathon, learning a new language, or writing a book. My friend, Hank, has successfully completed two Ironman triathlons. As you can imagine, his pre-Ironman training regimen was extremely physically and mentally strenuous. Undoubtedly, the physical output required to swim 2.4 miles, ride 112 miles on a bicycle, then run a 26.2-mile marathon without a break would create a massive outpouring of adrenaline and other stress hormones. But, unlike fleeing a predator for 12 consecutive hours, my friend experienced this grueling physical feat as transformative and exhilarating. Why? Because rather than being fearful or feeling victimized, he was empowered, focused, and motivated to succeed.

Distress, on the other hand, refers to a negative or aversive state in which an individual's coping and adaptation strategies fail to return her to physiological or psychological homeostasis (Selye 1956). In human terms, distress is experienced as suffering, anguish, or pain resulting from undesirable, uncontrollable, or difficult circumstances that tax a person's physical and emotional resources, such as natural disasters, divorce, death of a loved one, or an excessive workload. The extent to which we experience an event as distressing depends on its intensity, severity, duration, and controllability. For example, factors such as the magnitude of real or perceived threat, injury, loss of life, property damage, and whether the event elicited feelings of loss, shame, or humiliation can influence how we respond to, and recover from challenging circumstances. Likewise, genetic constitution, learning history, coping style, attitude, self-esteem, access to social support, and ability to find meaning in the face of adversity can impact resiliency.

Context can also affect our experience of stress. Individual factors such as the demands of parenting and family life, the presence of high conflict, poor communication, an excessive workload, economic pressures, disease, disability, or major psychological problems are all known to amplify the experience of stress. Likewise, environmental threats, such as an unsafe neighborhood, poverty, excess noise, violence, crime, environmental toxins, or political unrest can intensify the negativity of our experience (Benson 2000).

Distress and eustress differ biochemically, as seen by assessing the levels of two stress hormones, cortisol and dehydroepiandrosterone (DHEA), that are released by the adrenal glands when we experience stress. Cortisol converts fat and sugar into energy that the brain and body use when responding to threat. It also suppresses biological functions like digestion, growth, and reproduction. DHEA is a neurosteroid – a hormone that helps the brain process and recover from stressful experiences – that aids in learning, neuroplasticity, and growth (Boudarene, Legros, & Tilsit-Berthier 2001).

Both cortisol and DHEA are important for regulating body and brain function. When stress is chronically high, cortisol levels are elevated, increasing our risk for cardiovascular disease, suppressed immune function, and depression. On the other hand, when we engage in activities that cause eustress, DHEA levels are elevated, reducing the risk for anxiety, depression, heart disease, degenerative brain disorders, and other stress-related conditions. The ratio of cortisol to DHEA, often referred to as the growth index of the stress response, is a marker of whether stress is noxious or adaptive. A higher growth index reflects a greater amount of DHEA relative to cortisol. The higher the growth index, the more resilient to stress we are believed to be. Emerging research suggests that this growth index may be influenced by attitude. Specifically, the less stressful we perceive our lives to be, the more capable we feel, and the higher the growth index. This suggests that your experience of stress is determined, in part, by your mindset (Boudarene, Legros, & Tilsit-Berthier 2001).

Stress and the Brain

The Limbic System

The limbic system is located in the midbrain and includes parts the frontal, parietal, and temporal lobes. It consists of a complex array of highly interconnected structures including the thalamus, hypothalamus, amygdala, hippocampus, basal ganglia, and cingulate gyrus. The limbic system is often referred to as the "emotion" or "feeling and reacting" brain. It is intimately involved in interpreting stimuli via "bottom-up" processing (Figure 2.1). This means that information from the external environment is filtered through the brain's emotional circuitry prior to being projected to higher order "thinking" centers for interpretation. In real terms, bottom-up processing is what occurs when you react before weighing the circumstances of your behavior. For example, when a pedestrian steps in the path of your car, you slam on the brakes. It isn't until after an accident has been averted that you begin to interpret the details of the event (Gazzaniga, Ivry, & Mangun 2013).

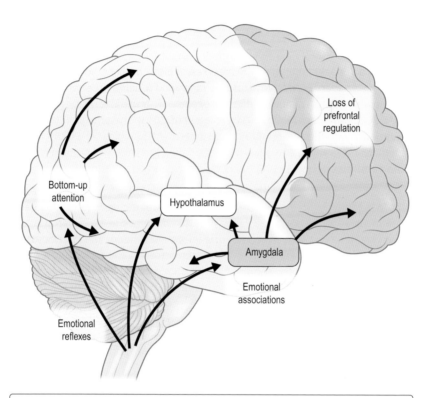

Bottom-up processing is a stimulus-driven strategy where perception begins at the level of sensory input. Sensory information is hierarchically processed and interpreted until pieces of information form a perceptible whole. Bottom-up processing emphasizes the salience of the stimulus. Stimuli that elicit emotional reactions, such as anxiety and fear, strengthen amygdala function, and inhibit higher-order abilities of the prefrontal cortex (PFC) such as working memory, attentional control, and emotion regulation. This results in a rapid, reflexive, emotional response.

Figure 2.1

Bottom-up processing and stress

Several limbic system structures are of particular importance when it comes to stress. The hypothalamus is a small structure situated under the thalamus, directly above the brainstem. It functions as a relay station, facilitating communication between the nervous and endocrine systems, and influencing the regulation of hormones that control a wide range of bodily functions including the stress response. From the instant danger is detected, the hypothalamus sends a chemical message to the adrenal glands, stimulating the production of adrenaline, norepinephrine and other stress hormones that rapidly flood into the bloodstream, supercharging the body's energy stores and increasing heart rate, respiration, blood pressure, and metabolism (Gazzaniga et al. 2013). In other words, it plays a key function in initiating the stress response.

The amygdala, located near the hypothalamus in the middle of the brain, is one of the most well-known limbic structures. It is responsible for encoding, processing, and storing of emotional information, and plays a pivotal function in emotional learning, processing emotional experience, affective expression, and the formation of memories associated with emotional events (Gazzaniga et al. 2013). The amygdala engages in a complex dance with the autonomic nervous system (ANS), which we will discuss below. Heightened activity of the amygdala has been linked to a variety of mood disturbances including anxiety, obsessive-compulsive disorders, and post-traumatic stress.

The hippocampus facilitates the consolidation of information from short-term to long-term memory, as well as spatial navigation. It is particularly sensitive to chronic stress, and plays an important role in stress resilience. The hippocampus aids in emotion regulation by relaying contextual information about the specific threat to the amygdala and prefrontal cortex (PFC), a structure in the frontal lobe that aids in the regulation of complex cognitive, emotional and behavioral functioning. This facilitates discrimination between threat and safety, allowing us to determine whether to remain in an alert state, or initiate a rest and recovery period. Emotion regulation is achieved when activity of the amygdala is balanced with that of the hippocampus and PFC. Chronic stress threatens that balance by overtaxing the systems responsible for mobilization and limiting the opportunity for rest, growth, and repair.

Like the hypothalamus, the amygdala and hippocampus are activated instantaneously once threat is detected. Because the limbic system is wired for survival, it can operate on an all-or-none principal, meaning that, once triggered, you are immediately primed for battle or retreat. As you will see in subsequent chapters, this state of reactivity doesn't always bode well for our relationships.

The Executive System

The executive system refers to a group of structures in the brain's frontal lobe that are responsible for "top-down" mental processes such as attentional control, organizing information, planning, impulse regulation, memory, problem solving, verbal reasoning and task switching (Gazzaniga et al. 2013) (Figure 2.2). "Top-down" refers to conceptually driven mental events that are influenced by internal cognitive factors like thoughts, expectations, values, and beliefs. In other words, when engaging in top-down processing we use existing knowledge and seek out information and experiences that "fill in the blanks." This allows us to use accumulated knowledge as a frame of reference, rather than figuring out each situation from scratch. For example, we draw on prior knowledge (and experience) that a rattlesnake is venomous, rather than sticking out our hand to see what happens if it bites us. Top-down processing also regulates emotions such as fear and anxiety. This occurs through the use of conscious coping mechanisms such as distraction, reappraisal of threat, emotional suppression, or unconscious processes that inhibit physiological arousal or that divert attention away from a threatening stimulus.

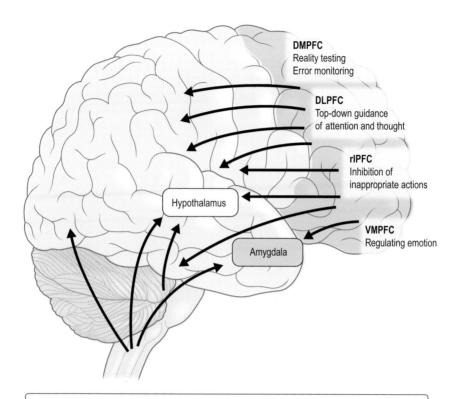

Top-down processing refers to conceptually driven mental events that are influenced by internal cognitive dimensions such as thoughts, feelings, expectations and beliefs. Existing knowledge is used to interpret current circumstances, allowing us to draw on prior knowledge to interpret an event. This form of processing relies on activation of structures in the prefrontal cortex (PFC) responsible for attention, inhibition, emotion regulation, reality testing, working memory, and other executive functions that enable planful responding. During stressful circumstances, the PFC and related functions are inhibited by the limbic system, decreasing the probability of utilizing conscious coping strategies.

Figure 2.2

Top-down processing and stress

The executive system is also associated with important social functions related to self-regulation and emotion-regulation, as well as some aspects of social and emotional intelligence (Goleman 2005). It allows us to use prior working knowledge of societal norms to determine how to behave in certain contexts and circumstances. For instance, most of us have learned that it isn't appropriate to have a loud conversation in a library. Knowing this, we modulate our behavior to accommodate the environment and those in it. In many respects, top-down processing is akin to exercising mindfulness. When behaving mindfully, we use a combination of attention, present-focused awareness, and prior knowledge to determine how we will relate to others. This is far different from a "bottom-up" approach where we react first and consider the consequences of our behavior later. Although the executive system is most often associated with adaptive strategies like planning and reasoning, it also has a downside. We can use its cognitive capacities to generate stories and relive memories that evoke strong emotional reactions like fear, terror, grief, anxiety and joy. As we will explore below, these mental events can trigger the stress response.

The limbic system, executive, and autonomic nervous system (ANS) are highly interconnected, with each sending millions of signals back and forth to encode, retrieve, organize, interpret, and remember incoming information, as well as to coordinate a response (Figure 2.3). As such, they participate in a mind–body "dance" in which each mutually inform and influence the other. This has important implications when we later consider how stress physiology can impair higher order cognitive capacities that we use to negotiate stressful situations.

The Autonomic Nervous System

The autonomic nervous system's (ANS) primary responsibility is to catalyze a response to environmental demands, and to maintain homeostatic balance during which rest, repair, and growth are possible (Llewellyn-Smith & Verberne 2011). The ANS is divided into two major branches: the sympathetic nervous system (SNS) and the parasympathetic nervous system (PNS) (Figure 2.4). The SNS is like a physiological "gas pedal." When an organism perceives threat, the SNS dumps a cascade of stress hormones into the bloodstream that

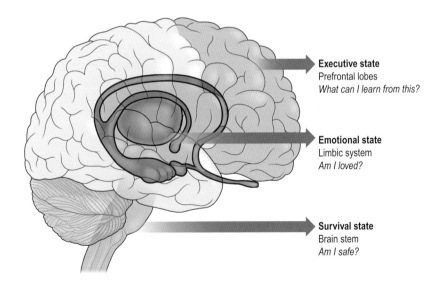

Executive state
Prefrontal lobes
What can I learn from this?

Emotional state
Limbic system
Am I loved?

Survival state
Brain stem
Am I safe?

Figure 2.3
Three brain states

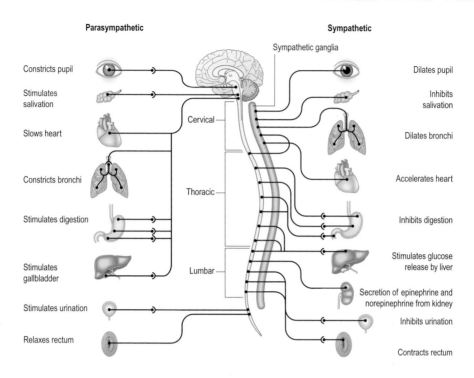

Parasympathetic

Sympathetic

Sympathetic ganglia

Constricts pupil

Dilates pupil

Stimulates salivation

Inhibits salivation

Cervical

Slows heart

Dilates bronchi

Constricts bronchi

Accelerates heart

Thoracic

Stimulates digestion

Inhibits digestion

Stimulates glucose release by liver

Stimulates gallbladder

Lumbar

Secretion of epinephrine and norepinephrine from kidney

Stimulates urination

Inhibits urination

Relaxes rectum

Contracts rectum

Figure 2.4

Autonomic nervous system (ANS)

increase heart rate, blood pressure and respiration, contract muscle, and depress all non-essential functions like digestion. In this state, the brain's fear circuitry, which resides in the limbic system, is also dominant, drawing important resources away from the executive system, including the prefrontal cortex and other cortical regions of the brain where planning, reasoning and effective communication occur. When the SNS is dominant and the executive system is inhibited, social behavior becomes limited, and we are more likely to resort to survival strategies such as aggression, avoidance or withdrawal.

The counterbalance to the SNS, the PNS, is often thought of as a physiological "brake pedal." Under conditions of threat, the PNS is inhibited. Conversely, in situations of safety, the PNS initiates the relaxation response, which depresses heart rate, blood pressure and respiration, reduces muscle tone/contraction, and allows the organism to engage in reparative and restorative functions (Everly & Lating 2013). In this state, the brain's fear circuitry is no longer mobilized, freeing up higher order, cognitive functioning and enabling a wider and more flexible range of thoughts, feelings, and behavior.

The Vagus Nerve and the Vagal System

The vagus nerve is an important part of the PNS. The word vagus is Latin for wandering. It travels through a great deal of the body, originating in the medulla oblongata in the brain stem and projecting to many visceral organs including the heart, lungs and digestive tract, independently of the spinal column (Figure 2.5). The vagal system represents a complex of nerve branches that relay signals from the brain to the body (efferent) and from visceral organs to the brain (afferent). This bi-directional communication allows for the efficient regulation of metabolic output in response to environmental demands (Porges 2011).

Activity of the vagus nerve is referred to as vagal tone, which is a reflection of the functional state of the ANS. It is measured by way of the amplitude of respiratory sinus

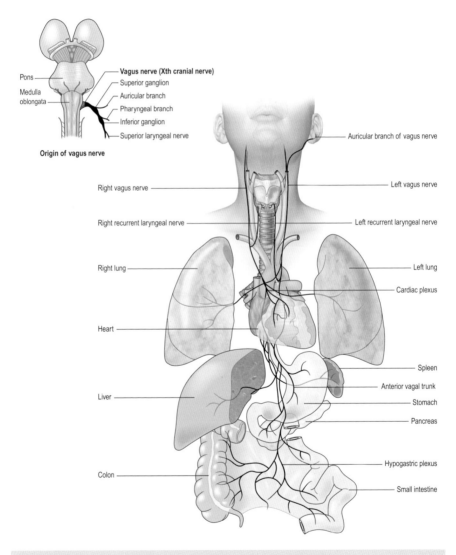

Figure 2.5

Vagus nerve

arrhythmia (RSA) variability. RSA variability is an indicator of heart rate variability, or the rhythmic increase and decrease in heart rate that naturally occurs as you inhale and exhale. This oscillation between acceleration and deceleration takes place due to the synchronous activation of the SNS and PNS. The SNS is associated with heart rate increase and the PNS with heart rate decrease.

The amplitude of RSA variability is considered a measure of vagal tone because it is an indication of the influence of the vagus nerve on the heart. Higher amplitude RSA variability suggests greater vagal tone. Greater vagal tone has been linked to a variety of positive health outcomes, including positive emotionality (Kok & Frederickson 2010), and an increased ability to respond effectively to stress and its increasing metabolic and environmental demands (Smeets 2010). In other words, higher vagal tone may serve as a protective factor against stress and stress-related illness. Emerging research suggests that a high vagal tone is associated with decreased emotional reactivity, enhanced empathic response, and higher levels of emotion regulation and psychological wellbeing. High vagal tone may also be predictive of short- and long-term prognosis in health conditions including dementia, cardiovascular disease, and even cancer prognosis (De Couck & Gidron 2013; De Couck, Mravec, & Gidron 2012; Gidron, De Couck, & De Greve 2014; Tsuji et al. 1996).

Vagal Tone and Social Behavior

Charles Darwin first noted the vagus nerve and its importance in social behavior in 1872. In his book, *The Expression of Emotions in Man and Animals* (Darwin 1872), he proposed that the central nervous system and the vagus nerve engage in a dynamic, mutual exchange of neurologic information that influences the spontaneous expression of emotion. Darwin contended that human affective expression is integral to survival and adaptation. Rather than being simply a reaction to experience, Darwin hypothesized that emotional expression is reciprocally linked to physiology, and that distinct neural pathways bi-directionally exchange information between brain structures and major visceral organs such as the heart, lungs, and gut. "When the heart is affected it reacts on the brain," wrote Darwin, "and the state of the brain again reacts through the pneumogastric (vagus) nerve on the heart; so that under any excitement there will be much mutual action and reaction between these, the two most important organs of the body" (Darwin 1872, p. 69). This is perhaps one of the first Western scientific acknowledgements of the mind–body connection!

Behavioral neuroscientist Stephen Porges and other contemporary neuroscientists and clinical researchers study the relationship between the vagus nerve and the development and maintenance of adaptive and maladaptive social functioning. In his book, *The Polyvagal Theory: Neurophysiological Foundations of Emotion, Attachment, Communication and Self-Regulation* (Porges 2011), Porges explored Polyvagal Theory, which details the phylogenic evolution of the human nervous system and the role of vagal tone in the development of social behavior (Table 2.1). Polyvagal Theory is predicated on the assumption that the human ANS is derived from three phylogenic stages of neurological development (Porges 2001, 2009, 2011).

TABLE 2.1
Polygenetic States of Vagus Development

Stage	ANS component	Behavioral function	Lower motor neurons
III	Myelinated vagus (ventral vagal complex)	Social communication, self-soothing and calming, inhibit "arousal"	Nucleus ambiguus
II	Sympathetic adrenal system	Mobilization (active avoidance)	Spinal cord
I	Unmyelinated vagus (dorsal vagal complex)	Immobilization (death feigning, passive avoidance)	Dorsal motor nucleus of the vagus

Phylogenic stages of the Polyvagal Theory From Biol Psychol. 2007 Feb; 74(2):116–143

The first stage, which we see in primitive life forms, is associated with immobilization behaviors such as freezing and feigning death in the presence of threat. The second stage includes SNS influence, which increases metabolic output and inhibits PNS/vagal tone to mobilize for fight or flight. The third stage, which is unique to mammals, includes the addition of myelinated vagal nerves that are capable of rapidly regulating cardiac output to facilitate both engagement and disengagement from environmental stimuli.[1] This myelinated branch of the vagal system controls facial muscles associated with speaking, swallowing, sucking, and, most importantly, breathing. It also regulates SNS pathways to the heart and can rapidly initiate relaxation and calm. These regulatory systems of the vagus and associated cranial nerves are believed to provide the substrate for emotional experiences and social behavior.

Polyvagal Theory (Porges 2001, 2009, 2011) links the evolution of the autonomic nervous system to emotional experience and expression, vocal communication and social behavior. In his decades of research examining the ways in which the phylogenic development of the vagus has affected human behavioral expression, Porges found that the more recently evolved, myelinated branches of the vagus nerve found in mammals play a distinct role in attention, self-regulation, communication, emotional expression, resilience to stress and other capacities central to social functioning. These myelinated vagus fibers, which send signals to the brain much more quickly than the phylogenically older, unmyelinated fibers, inhibit these older systems. As a result, the newer, myelinated vagal system in mammals can override the signals of the SNS, a phenomenon that Porges refers to as the vagal brake.

The vagal brake's essential function is to regulate heart rate through the rapid inhibition and disinhibition of vagal tone to the heart. When the brake is applied, vagal tone increases and cardiac output is reduced, promoting relaxation, self-soothing, growth, and repair. Conversely, when the brake is released and the SNS becomes dominant,

---

1   Myelin refers to a white, fatty substance that surrounds the axon of certain nerve cells. This layer, the myelin sheath, electrically insulates nerve fibers from other electrically charged molecules, increasing their rate of signal transmission when compared to unmyelinated nerves.

heart rate increases and the organism is mobilized to address environmental demands. When the vagal brake is inhibited, phylogenically older autonomic responses are utilized, resulting in a narrowed repertoire of fight or flight behaviors in response to threat.

Proponents of Polyvagal Theory assert that the vagal brake plays a central role in the development of appropriate social behavior. Because of its capacity to rapidly depress or recruit the SNS in response to environmental demands, the brake allows for immediate engagement and disengagement with others during social interaction. Although Polyvagal Theory requires considerably more empirical support before it gains wide acceptance, it offers an interesting perspective from which to consider the influence of the mind–body relationship on interpersonal dynamics.

We do know that vagal tone and the PNS play an important role in social behavior including regulating facial and emotional expression and communication (Beauchaine 2001; Berntson, Sarter, & Cacioppo 2003: Porges 2009, 2011). Numerous studies with infants and young children show that vagal tone is an important indicator of self-regulation, sustained attention, resiliency and the ability to self-soothe after experiencing a stressor (e.g. Porges 1992, 1996; Porges, Doussard-Roosevelt, & Maiti 1994; Porges et al. 1996). This capacity to regulate behavior is a critically important function in relationship. Those who are able to think and act flexibly, maintain attentional control, and regulate emotions and behaviors are far more able to respond appropriately to interpersonal stressors and demands than those who lack these competencies.

The vagus nerve operates bi-directionally, both sending and receiving signals between the brain and visceral organs (Yuan & Silberstein 2015a, 2015b, 2016). When the body experiences physical or psychological stress, the vagus is recruited in the initiation of a compensatory behavioral response by either applying or releasing the vagal brake. But when real or perceived stress is chronic, homeostatic balance is difficult, if not impossible to maintain. The SNS becomes consistently dominant, and the vagal brake is less frequently applied. Persistent SNS dominance leaves the system in a constant state of stress, increasing the risk for physical and emotional illness.

As mentioned above, the vagus nerve controls muscles associated with speaking, swallowing, sucking, and, most importantly, breathing (Porges 2011). It is inherently linked to social behavior through its activation of the muscles of the face and neck including those that influence facial expression and vocal resonance. Research suggests that higher vagal tone and the capacity to effectively use the vagal brake are associated with greater emotional stability, cognitive flexibility, behavioral regulation, prosody of speech, and appropriate facial expression – all key capacities of socially-skilled behavior. Conversely, poor vagal brake regulation is linked to affective and behavioral dysfunction (Porges 2011).

In addition to the innervation of facial muscles, the vagus controls and is influenced by respiration. When the vagal brake is activated and the PNS system is recruited, heart and respiration rates lower. Conversely, when the brake is lifted and the SNS dominates, respiration and heart rate become rapid and survival-oriented behaviors dominate.

The vagus nerve also influences, and is influenced by, functioning of the major viscera, including the heart, gut, and lungs. Of these, respiration (lung activity), is the only visceral function that we can easily and consciously control (Brown & Gerbarg 2009; Gerbarg & Brown 2015). This means that the vagus nerve can be influenced by consciously manipulating the breath. As you will recall from our prior discussion of RSA oscillation during the breath cycle, vagal tone (and PNS activity) increases during exhalation. By slowing down our rate of respiration and elongating our exhalation, we can activate the vagal brake, and volitionally elicit the relaxation response. Once this response is initiated and the PNS is dominant, we cease to be governed by the brain's fear circuitry that limits our capacity to effectively think, plan, reason and respond to others (Brown & Gerbarg 2012). This means we are no longer subject to a narrow range of thoughts, feelings, and perceptions or limited to defensive or escape behaviors (Brown & Gerbarg 2012). In other words, intentional breathing decreases the stress response and increases cognitive and behavioral flexibility, which enhances our ability to be mindfully present in relationships.

The Psychophysiology of Stress in Relationships

Dr. John Gottman, a renowned psychologist and marriage researcher, is the author of several influential books, including *The Seven Principles for Making Marriage Work* (Gottman & Silver 1999). Gottman first gained national attention in 1998 after publishing an article in the *Journal of Marriage and Family* in which he and his colleagues were able to predict divorce with 83% accuracy (Gottman et al. 1998). In the study, newlywed couples were videotaped discussing a contentious topic for 15 minutes. These tapes were then viewed and behaviors including criticism, defensiveness, avoidance, and contempt were coded. Gottman and his colleagues hypothesized that these negative behaviors would predict divorce three to six years later. They were right 83% of the time.

Based on this research, Gottman and his team isolated four key factors that predicted marital breakdown, which they named the "Four Horsemen of the Apocalypse." These include criticizing a partner's personality, contempt (acting from a position of superiority), defensiveness, and stonewalling, or withdrawal from interaction. Studies consistently show that the overwhelming majority of couples who demonstrate these behaviors end up divorced (Gottman & Silver 1999).

Some of Gottman's observational research took place in a mock studio apartment complete with video cameras often referred to as "The Love Lab." The "lab" was designed to document couples as they interacted during everyday circumstances – sort of a researcher's version of reality TV. To make the experience as life-like as possible, couples were instructed to bring their pets, groceries, laptops, hobbies, and whatever else would help to mimic a typical weekend. The couples were fitted with electrodes to measure physiological indicators of stress, such as heart rate and respiration, to assess whether physiological changes influenced their ability to communicate, particularly during stressful encounters.

Many years of observing and monitoring hundreds of couples led to a groundbreaking discovery about stress and communication. During stressful conversations we experience "flooding" – a physiological reaction characterized by sensations like a racing heart, sweating, flushed face, and upset stomach. When we are "flooded," our heart speeds up to more than 100 beats per minute, blood pressure escalates and adrenaline is released. This is a clear sign that SNS arousal has taken over and that the limbic system, or emotional brain, is governing behavior (Gottman & Silver 1999).

When it comes to marriage, flooding can predict disaster. "Recurring episodes of flooding lead to divorce for two reasons," Gottman says. "First, they signal that at least one partner feels severe emotional distress when dealing with the other. Second, the physical sensations of feeling flooded – the increased heart rate, sweating, and so on – makes it virtually impossible to have a productive, problem-solving discussion. When the body goes into overdrive during an argument, it is responding to a very primitive alarm system we inherited from our prehistoric ancestors. Your ability to process information is reduced, meaning it's harder to pay attention to what your partner is saying. Creative problem solving goes out the window. You're left with the most reflexive, least intellectually sophisticated responses in your repertoire: to fight or flee. Any chance of resolving the issue is gone" (Gottman & Silver 1999, pp. 36–37). In fact, Gottman can reliably predict divorce just by looking at individuals' physiological readings during a tense conversation.

This doesn't just apply to marriage. Any difficult encounter with another person can lead to flooding. When in this state, it is difficult, if not impossible, to hear what others are trying to communicate. Because we feel threatened, we act out of self-preservation, unable to speak clearly or listen effectively. Flooding is a clear sign that we have lost our capacity to communicate skillfully.

In *The Seven Principles for Making Marriage Work*, John Gottman recommends taking a minimum of a 20-minute break to reset the system when feeling flooded (Gottman & Silver 1999). Although this is wise advice, there are circumstances, like business meetings and other public situations, when the luxury of taking time out doesn't exist. This is where the first step of the BREATHE model, intentional breathing, is particularly useful. The breath can be used as a tool to rapidly defuse the stress response before resorting to behaviors that we may regret later. As we will explore in Part II, the BREATHE model offers simple, accessible tools for de-escalating stress physiology and regaining a calm mind and body. These skills reduce SNS reactivity, increase awareness, and create space to interrupt the cycle of automatic, reactive behaviors that occur when we are chronically stressed and overwhelmed.

EXERCISE
How Stressed Do You Feel?

The following is a survey, The Perceived Stress Scale (Cohen, Kamarck, & Mermelstein 1983), which assesses your current level of stress. Take a few moments to complete the questions. What did you learn?

The questions in this scale ask you about your feelings and thoughts during the last month. In each case, please choose the number from 0–4 that reflects how often you felt or thought a certain way.

0 = Never, 1 = Almost never, 2 = Sometimes, 3 = Fairly often, 4 = Very often

1. In the last month, how often have you been upset because of something that happened unexpectedly?

2. In the last month, how often have you felt that you were unable to control the important things in your life?

3. In the last month, how often have you felt nervous and "stressed?"

4. In the last month, how often have you felt confident about your ability to handle your personal problems?

5. In the last month, how often have you felt that things were going your way?

6. In the last month, how often have you found that you could not cope with all the things that you had to do?

7. In the last month, how often have you been able to control irritations in your life?

8. In the last month, how often have you felt that you were on top of things?

9. In the last month, how often have you been angered because of things that were outside of your control?

10. In the last month, how often have you felt difficulties were piling up so high that you could not overcome them?

3 | Why Manage Chronic Stress?

Until you make the unconscious conscious, it will direct your life and you will call it fate.

C.G. Jung

Chronic stress kills. It not only harms your body, mind, and spirit, but your relationships as well. Research over the past several decades shows that high levels of persistent stress increase the risk for physical and psychological illness and dementia (Johansson et al. 2010; Kemeny 2003; Lupien et al. 2009; Kendler, Karkowsky & Prescott 1999; McCormick & Mathews 2007; Persson & Skoog 1996; Roozendaal, McEwen, & Chattarji 2009; Schneiderin, Ironson, & Siegel 2005; Selye 1956; Shaw & Krause 2002; Stawski et al. 2006; Yehuda et al. 2005). In spite of this, many of us continue to live high-pressure lives. We wear our stress like a badge of courage, reciting endless lists of to-dos with pride. When someone asks, "How are you?" we respond, "I've been working 60 hours a week," as if that were a good thing. We take on more than we can realistically handle, ignoring the toxic effects of our decisions. Then, one day we face a health scare, stare divorce in the face, or lose our job, and the tenuousness of our lifestyles becomes clear. When we live in a state of chronic stress, we suffer, as do others.

Suzanne is a 40-year-old advertising executive and single mother of two energetic school-aged girls. The daughter of a disabled mother and an alcoholic father, Suzanne put herself through college, always priding herself on her discipline, independence, and ability to thrive under tough conditions. At work, she is known for her creativity, ingenuity, keen problem solving, and for meeting and exceeding her clients' expectations. She's always at the top of her game and has had a meteoric rise to an upper level management position.

Recently, Suzanne learned that the agency where she works was sold to a large multinational corporation. In spite of her remarkable track record and tireless years of dedication, her job is now in jeopardy. Scores of highly paid colleagues have already been laid off or terminated as part of a new corporate restructuring plan, and Suzanne worries that she may be next.

As breadwinner and primary caregiver, Suzanne is wracked with fear, terrified by the possibility of losing her job and being unable to provide for her girls. She spends many sleepless nights running scores of scenarios through her mind. She meets each day with crippling anxiety and fatigue. Usually a doting mom, Suzanne now has little patience for her daughters' needs, often hiding her tears after snapping at them. Her outgoing personality has faded, leaving her feeling like a shell of her former self.

Fifty-nine-year-old Tal grew up in inner city Baltimore in the 1960s. His stooped, lanky six-foot frame bends under the weight of the world he carries squarely on his shoulders, the burden of struggle deeply etched into his brow. He is a welder and his wife, Ruth, is a housekeeper. Together they raised three thriving sons and a daughter through tough economic and political times. Much of their 36 years of marriage has been devoted to their church and to instilling the values of hard work and family in their now-grown children, each of whom is raising a family of their own.

The many years of struggle have left fault lines in the foundation of Tal and Ruth's marriage. He no longer has the energy to deal with her demands, often retreating to the television after a long workday. Ruth worries that her husband has lost interest and plans to leave her. Her fear comes out in critical fits of rage during which she accuses Tal of being lazy and doing too little around the house, even though she knows better. Tal, in turn, walks out, not returning home until well after midnight. He sleeps on the sofa.

Yolanda is a top executive at an emerging social media giant in Silicon Valley. As the daughter of successful and supportive parents, she has always been driven to please them. Her hard work ethic and fearless drive resulted in her graduating at the top of her class at Stanford and excelling in an MBA program at Harvard, where her professors showered her with accolades and helped her land her first prestigious position at a tech firm.

At barely 30 years of age, Yolanda has achieved remarkable success. Failure has never been part of her vocabulary and she is used to being loved and appreciated by all who surround her – until now. In spite of her strong academic credentials, Yolanda has little experience managing teams of people. She feels growing dissent among her staff and chooses to avoid tension and conflict rather than address it directly. She is terrified that her inexperience will be revealed, and she will lose her prominent position. She compensates for her fear and inexperience by allowing her supervisees to do whatever they want with very little guidance or accountability.

At first, this seemed to be a workable strategy; however, her staff's motivation and productivity have declined and her superiors are demanding results. In response, Yolanda has adopted a new management strategy: she calls frequent meetings where she channels her anxiety into berating her team and threatening them in an attempt to motivate them to work harder. When staff express the need for clear direction, she retaliates, accusing them of being incompetent. This month alone, three employees have resigned and another two have requested to be transferred to a different department. Yolanda now works 16-hour days, no longer exercising or spending time with friends or family to mollify her anxiety. She has asked her doctor for medication to deal with her "nerves" and to help her to sleep.

Suzanne, Tal, and Yolanda do their best to cope with high levels of chronic stress. Even though they each possess a great deal of strength and resilience, they find themselves overwhelmed and unable to meet the demands of their lives, work, and loved ones. For Suzanne, the persistent threat of losing her job has triggered historical insecurities around not having her fundamental needs met. The intense demands of her job and the high expectations that she has created for herself as a professional and as a mother have become more than she can bear, as she perceives her life falling apart. She reacts to her fear by retreating at work and lashing out in anger at home. This has left her feeling like a failure – an experience that she has worked to avoid at all costs.

Tal has always been the family bedrock, working tirelessly for decades at a strenuous job to keep a roof over his family's head, put food on the table, and give his children every opportunity that he could afford. At age 59, he finds himself exhausted, struggling to cope with a broken marriage and his growing feelings of anger and despair.

Yolanda has always been a superstar in her family's eyes and struggled mightily to be a high achiever. She is terrified that she will fail, not only embarrassing herself, but upsetting her parents as well. Her lifetime mantra of perfection-at-all-costs has left her feeling alone, isolated, and afraid to confide in anyone or ask for help. She is convinced that if she works harder she will make up for her lack of management experience; however, this fear-based strategy has left her on the verge of burnout.

Chronic Stress and the Mind

Suzanne, Tal, and Yolanda are each living life from a place of fear. Not only that, but the chronic stress that has characterized each of their lives has left them feeling unable to cope with personal and relationship demands and responsibilities. Fear and stress are useful and adaptive in moderation. Without them, our ancestors would have succumbed to predators, starvation, inhospitable climates, and natural disasters ages ago. However, when stress, anxiety, and fear are chronic, they can be debilitating.

Part of why we experience challenge as scary or stressful is a matter of mindset – the set of assumptions that we carry that affect our perceptions and behavior (Dweck 2007). When we frame our circumstances as menacing, we experience them as stressful. Conversely, when we see tests of our ability as growth opportunities, we are more likely to mobilize our physical and mental resources and make the most of the situation. In other words, our appraisal or interpretation of an event has considerable bearing on how stressful we experience it to be (Lazarus 1999; Semmer, McGrath, & Beehr 2005).

Our minds can both contribute to stress resilience and function as stress generators. In his groundbreaking book, *Why Zebras Don't Get Ulcers*, Robert Sapolsky pointed to an important difference between how humans and animals experience stress (Sapolsky 1998). For animals like a zebra, danger is often immediate and life threatening. A zebra sees a lion running straight for him and runs for his life. He will either succeed or be killed – end of story. Humans, on the other hand, have the capacity to recall the experience of being chased in exquisite detail. We can conjure up an image of the lioness and her gleaming fangs and imagine an endless string of scenarios. In other words, our minds keep the stress response alive by mentally recreating the past and ruminating about the future. From a physiological perspective, our brains and nervous systems don't know the difference. That's why we can experience intense physiological and emotional arousal just by imagining situations when we feel angry, hurt, aggressive, or fearful.

For many, mentally generated, fear-based scenarios cause a great deal of stress and anxiety. Like Yolanda, Tal, and Suzanne, we may obsess about failing loved ones, losing a job or a home, or ending a marriage. We may harbor fear about larger social issues like economic collapse, increasing crime rates, or even climate change. Regardless of how you generate psychological stress, what is important to remember is that your brain and body experience threat as a stressor, whether you come across danger directly or create scenarios in your mind. It's all the same.

Many of us remain stuck in a chronic stress cycle because we have difficulty prioritizing ourselves. We see self-care as being selfish or self-centered. Selfishness involves acting to satisfy our desires to the detriment of others. Self-care entails addressing our essential needs and health so that we can be present for ourselves and others. It's like putting on your oxygen mask first before helping the person next to you on an airplane. Even though it may seem heroic to sacrifice your needs for another, you can hurt those you love when you don't take time to care for yourself. The only person capable of changing that is you.

My friend Evan is a good example. He is a kind, loving, and dutiful son who devotes a good deal of time and energy caring for his elderly parents. He has spent the past three years driving hundreds of miles a week to tend to his ailing father while simultaneously caring for his mother and trying to hold down a full time job. Earlier this year, his father's health began to decline, so Evan reduced his work to part-time to spend more time shuttling his dad to doctor visits. This placed a great deal of physical and financial stress on Evan, but he believed that his duty to his family outweighed his commitment to himself. Several months later, he found himself in the emergency room after numerous bouts of intense chest pain. His blood pressure was elevated, he had put on weight, and he was exhausted. That was Evan's wake up call. In spite of his noble intention to care for his family, he was faced with the very clear reality that the very same nobility was killing him. Something had to change or his parents might outlive him.

Why Manage Chronic Stress?

Table 3.1 illustrates that eustress and chronic distress affect the body and mind in very different ways. Whereas eustress can increase energetic resources, heighten attention and awareness, and support rapid recovery and healing following a stressor, prolonged distress can deplete energy stores, cause chronic inflammation, hypertension, and increase the likelihood of psychological dysregulation (Selye 1956).

Allostasis refers to an organism's ability to adapt in the face of a stressful challenge (McEwen 1998; Sterling & Eyer 1988; Logan & Barksdale 2008). Allostatic load refers to "the price the body pays for being forced to adapt to adverse psychosocial or physical situations… it represents either the presence of too much stress, or the inefficient operation of the stress hormone response system, which must be turned on and then turned off again after the stressful situation is over" (McEwen 2000, p. 111). For example, hypertension (high blood pressure) is a chronic symptom of high allostatic load that forces the heart to work harder. It is a leading risk factor for cardiovascular diseases including stroke and heart attack. High allostatic load also affects the brain and the immune system, raising the number of immune cells in the blood stream and increasing the risk for systemic inflammation. Although inflammation is adaptive in the short term, neither the brain nor the immune system benefit from continuous, intense activation or high allostatic load (McEwen 2000). Chronic inflammation manifests as redness, swelling, joint pain and stiffness, and is associated with numerous serious illnesses including rheumatoid, psoriatic, and gouty arthritis. It is also related to autoimmune dysfunction including celiac disease, type 1 diabetes, Graves' disease, inflammatory bowel disease (IBD), and multiple sclerosis (MS).

TABLE 3.1

Positive and Negative Physical and Psychological Outcomes of Acute and Chronic Sympathetic Nervous System (SNS) Activation

Physical and psychological responses	Eustress – positive outcomes of stress	Distress – negative outcomes of chronic stress
Cortisol/adrenaline released into bloodstream	Mobilizes visceral organs and skeletal muscle for action	Physiological burnout, adrenal fatigue/failure
Sugar released from liver	Increases energy resources	Depletes energy resources
Heart rate acceleration	Mobilizes physical resources, to respond to challenge.	Heart disease
Blood vessel constriction		Hypertension
Respiration acceleration	Increased delivery of oxygen to the blood stream	SNS dominance/ respiratory disease
Muscle contraction	Prepares muscles for action	Chronic musculoskeletal pain
Digestion diversion of blood flow	Focuses resources to respond to challenge.	Digestive disorders (e.g. acid reflux, irritable bowel syndrome (IBS))
Heightened immune response	Supports rapid recovery and healing	Chronic systemic inflammation/ autoimmune disease (arthritis, IBS, fibromyalgia, cardiopulmonary disease)
Closure of bladder sphincter	Limit unnecessary bodily function	Urinary dysfunction
Diversion of blood flow away from sex organs		Sexual dysfunction
Heightened cognitive and emotional acuity and vigilance	Increases attention, motivation, awareness as well as pro-social and affiliative behavior	Psychological distress, rumination, reactivity, poor regulation of cognition, emotion and behavior, anxiety and depressive disorders, social withdrawal, relationship stress

Chronic stress is also linked to poor psychological health (Kendler, Karkowski, & Prescott 1999; Lupien et al. 2009; McEwen 2000). Studies show that persistent stress presents a major risk for depression and anxiety disorders, post-traumatic stress disorder (PTSD), eating disorders like anorexia nervosa and bulimia, increased alcohol and drug consumption, and substance abuse. This is, in part, because chronic stress alters brain circuitry by increasing the functioning of the amygdala, while simultaneously inhibiting the hippocampus and prefrontal cortex (PFC), the latter of which plays a significant role in emotion regulation, and modulation of the stress response (Arnstein 1999, 2016; Lupien et al. 2009; Roozendaal et al. 2009).

A scientific review published in *Current Opinions in Psychiatry* examined neuroimaging studies of anxiety and stress in healthy and clinical populations, and the neurocircuitry and brain structures most impacted by chronic stress exposure. These structures included the amygdala, which plays a key role in emotional processing, the prefrontal cortex (PFC), which is associated with cognitive appraisal and emotion regulation, and the hippocampus, which governs long-term memory and spatial navigation. The review found consistent evidence of increased amygdala activation and reduced PFC function in chronically stressed individuals. This pattern reflected a tendency toward greater anxiety and negative affect due to a reduced ability to regulate mood. These stress-induced brain changes also posed a risk for psychological disorders and dementia (Mah, Szabuniewicz, & Fiocco 2016). In a 35-year longitudinal study of a community sample of 1,462 women aged 39–60 years, the risk of dementia, particularly Alzheimer's disease, was considerably higher among those who reported experiencing stress during at least one of the five assessment points (Johansson et al. 2010). This parallels prior research that documents stressful life events and PTSD as risk factors for cognitive decline and dementia (Greenberg et al. 2014; Persson & Skoog 1996).

Some of the most compelling evidence as to why we need to reduce chronic stress is neurobiological. Vulnerability to stress is particularly acute during critical periods of prenatal developmental, in the months following birth, in early childhood, and again in adolescence. During these intervals, important neural pathways are developed and pruned that set the stage for a lifetime of cognitive and behavioral strategies for coping with life stress (Gunnar & Quevedo 2007; Lupien et al. 2009; Kasatsoreos & McEwen 2013).

In 2013, neuroscientists Ilia Karatsoreos and Bruce McEwen published a review of research examining the neurobiological and psychophysiological effects of stress on development across the lifespan (Kasatsoreos & McEwen 2013). They reported that adverse childhood experiences have long-term consequences on resilience and psychological wellbeing, but that neural circuits can, to some degree, be "rewired." This neuroplasticity, the ability to revise or establish new neural networks, persists throughout our lives. Although we do not know the extent to which neuroplasticity and positive life-experience can reverse the effects of stress or contribute to increased resilience, the good news is that the brain is capable of repairing itself, but only when chronic stress ceases (Bremner 2005; Everly & Lating 2013).

Chronic Stress and Relationships

In addition to its effect on individuals, chronic stress can be detrimental to relationships. In two separate studies, psychologists Neff and Karney (2009) asked couples to complete daily diaries for a week in addition to completing questionnaires regarding their marital satisfaction, aspects of their relationship, self-esteem, and attachment styles (relationship closeness, anxiety, and independence). The first study included 146 newlywed couples assessed over seven days. The second followed 82 newlywed couples for four years. Both studies showed that couples, particularly wives, experiencing high levels of stress were more likely to have negative reactions to the daily ups and downs of their relationships. These findings persisted independently of their reported self-esteem and attachment style. Interestingly, a husband or wife's individual relationship skills did not correlate with his or her ability to respond effectively to a spouse in the presence of high levels of stress. This suggests that even those with strong relationship skills faltered in the presence of high levels of stress, most likely because it led to them to evaluate their relationships negatively (Neff & Karney 2009).

The effects of chronic stress are circular. When we're stressed, ill, unhappy, or our relationships are failing, we tend to feel more stressed. The more stressed we feel, the more likely we are to become ill and feel strain in our relationships. Do you ever feel as though, no matter how hard you work or what you do, you are usually falling behind or unable to please everyone? Are you frequently ill, exhausted, frustrated, angry, irritable, sad, anxious, or overwhelmed? These are just a few of the signs that you're running on the hamster wheel of chronic stress. You're not alone. Our society is built on a tenuous foundation of stressed-out people doing their best to cope with persistent overwhelm. But there's something that you can do about it. You can learn to take care of yourself.

The Importance of Awareness

As mentioned earlier, a high-stress lifestyle tends to be a twenty-first century norm. Because of this, and the fact that we are surrounded by fellow travelers who are also stressed out, we tend to normalize persistent stress, often diminishing or dismissing its effects. If we're all doing it, chronic stress doesn't seem so unusual. We commiserate about it with our friends, on social media, or around the office. We tell ourselves that everyone is stressed, so there's no use complaining about it.

Sometimes we get a glimpse of the effects of chronic stress when something isn't working. But it can be difficult to pay attention or identify the source of that discomfort when we're juggling competing priorities. In fact, examining the sources of stress in our lives can feel like another stressor, so we may feel compelled to press on and maintain the status quo. When under pressure, it is also difficult to maintain focus. A study of 2,250 American adult men and women found that many of us are walking around distracted (Killingsworth & Gilbert 2010). Participants were asked to complete a series of questions about how they were feeling, what they were doing, and whether they were thinking about something other than what they were doing. Forty-six percent of respondents reported frequent mind wandering regardless of what they were doing, and indicated being less happy when their minds were off task than when they weren't. Remarkably, what participants were thinking predicted their happiness more than what they were doing, suggesting that our mood may be more influenced by our thoughts than our actions. This led the study's authors to conclude, "A human mind is a wandering mind, and a wandering mind is an unhappy mind" (Killingsworth & Glibert 2010, p. 932).

One of the first orders of business in becoming aware of and attuned to your stress level is to understand how the mind, body, and brain process stress. In Chapters 2 and 3 we reviewed what occurs in the body and brain. In the next chapter, we will explore the workings of the mind, and see how the stories we tell ourselves can enhance or impair health, happiness, and relationship success.

4 | The Stories We Tell: Why Mindset Matters

The words you speak become the house you live in.

Hafiz

Your beliefs become your thoughts. Your thoughts become your words. Your words become your actions. Your actions become your habits. Your habits become your values. Your values become your destiny.

Gandhi

When I first met Joel, he was a 57-year-old environmental scientist who had worked at the same government agency for over 30 years. He was suffering from depression and social isolation and had few supportive relationships. Joel reported feeling unbearably lonely, not to mention angry and resentful of all of the people who had let him down. He was convinced that no one liked him. He related stories of a lifetime of feeling left out, criticized, and alienated by family members and colleagues. By living out the story that no one liked him, he had manifested the one thing that he feared most – being alone.

Joel had been a loner as long as he could remember. He had very few friends and spent the majority of his time reading history books and fantasizing about flying planes. While the other boys were playing sports and chasing girls, Joel hid in the shadows. He struggled awkwardly with conversations, often making comments that were tangential or irrelevant. Most of his classmates and peers felt him to be odd and ill at ease, and they avoided him. Although he was never bullied, he moved through life in obscurity, navigating a world of his own making. He told himself that he was disliked, misunderstood, and that people were making fun of him and he grew more angry and resentful as time wore on. The more rigid his narrative, the more reclusive he became. He adopted a mask of indifference that kept people at bay, all to avoid the pain of rejection.

Joel hadn't always felt so hopeless. When he finished graduate school and began working a mid-level professional position, he was riding the wave of being a top-notch student and was enthusiastic about his career and future. But this high was short lived. As soon as he entered the workforce, he immediately began having problems. His supervisors continuously reprimanded him for not meeting deadlines. Convinced that they didn't like him, he tried to gain their favor by taking on extra projects and over-time shifts. This only served to garner the attention of his co-workers, who accused him of sucking up to management and ostracized him. In response, he alienated himself from others even more.

Joel's belief that no one likes him has taken a heavy toll. He feels that no one listens to his ideas or gives him credit for his work. He responds to requests with shoulder shrugs or curt remarks, giving the impression that he is self-important, uncooperative, and periodically bursts out during staff meetings, accusing his peers of stealing his ideas or being idiots. Even though Joel worked hard and successfully passed exams that should have resulted in promotion, his inability to relate to others has kept him stuck in virtually the same position for decades. He has given up on career advancement, convincing himself that he is content in his current dead end job as long as he is left alone to do his work.

Joel's problems don't end at the office. The story that no one likes him dominates his life. His marriage of nearly 30 years has been riddled with periods of bitter fighting and the threat of divorce. His wife is intensely frustrated by his intolerance, overly controlling, passive aggressive behavior and inability to communicate with her and their grown children. His children treat him with disrespect, making fun of him and his odd ways. Most of the time, he feels miserable and alone.

Joel is an example of someone whose personal story has shaped his life. He has little ability to differentiate himself from it and finds evidence that no one likes him with nearly everyone he meets. Recognizing our stories and how they influence how we respond and relate to others is a hallmark of becoming self-aware and a cornerstone of mindfulness. But it can be difficult to discriminate ourselves from our stories unless we are conscious of them and can understand where they came from.

Developing Personal Narratives

Humans are natural storytellers. We organize our internal worlds using language, spending a great proportion of our time encoding information into matrices of meaning that we use to interpret and predict social events, relationship experiences, and outcomes (Boroditsky 2011; Hayes, Blackledge, & Barnes-Holmes 2001; Holtgraves & Kashima 2008; Pennebaker, Mehl, & Niederhoffer 2003). Even now, you are probably mentally describing your reaction to the last sentence. Whether via writing, music, art, dance, or other forms of expression, communication and language are an integral part of the human experience.

We have a social imperative to connect with each other and to make sense of the world we inhabit. It is part of our evolutionary heritage. We started by drawing lines in the sand, etching cave paintings, carving bone and wood figures, and moved on from there. Stories have been used for millennia by indigenous cultures to convey everything from hunting wisdom to navigation, to passing on values and traditions. They are as central to our identities as the names that we have been given (Konner 2011).

Notice the next time you find yourself sitting in traffic, riding a subway or bus, or waiting in line. Chances are you'll find yourself knee deep in a story. It may be recounting a newspaper article you read over morning coffee, making plans for the weekend, or re-hashing a disagreement. Either way, it's a story, and it is likely that one is running somewhere through your mind even as you read this. That's some pretty advanced multitasking!

We begin to create stories very early in life. Developmental psychologist Jean Piaget, most well-known for his four stages of child cognitive development, proposed that children are like "little scientists" who conduct an ongoing and endless series of tests to try to make sense of the world. Between roughly the ages of two and seven, children are in what Piaget called the "preoperational stage" (Piaget 1936). During this stage, children engage in a continuous stream of pretend play where they try on roles in an attempt to see what fits. If you observe them closely, you will notice that they often narrate their play with elaborate stories.

Children are also masterful at exploring different identities. While at play, they can shape shift from one character to another seamlessly. My former neighbor's three-year-old son, Tyler, is an excellent example. He is often immersed in pretend play, transforming himself from a bird to a dinosaur to a malevolent dictator all in the span of an hour. What's amazing is that he not only tries on roles but also keenly observes adults' reactions. The responses that children receive from others have strong bearing on their emerging identities and perceptions of what works interpersonally and what doesn't. They try on different roles and experiment with different archetypes (e.g. the good child, the domineering child, the pleaser, the athlete, or the mischief maker) while simultaneously and often unconsciously collecting copious amounts of data.

Early twentieth century sociologist Charles Cooley deemed this phenomenon "the looking-glass self" (Cooley 1998). According to his theory, children's identities are formed based on interpersonal interactions and their perceptions of how they are received by others. He proposed that our self-concept is shaped in three ways: by imagining how we appear to others, by judging how we believe others see us, and by creating a self based on how we think we are being viewed.

Tyler is the looking-glass self in action. One day while walking my dog with a friend, we ran into him and his mom, Nancy, in front of their home. Nancy announced that today Tyler was a bird, at which point he began to flap his bent elbows like scrawny wings and let out a series of ear-piercing squawks. Even though I enjoy Tyler immensely, that day his squawks could have shattered glass. My friend and I excused ourselves and hurried off.

On the way back from walking our dogs, some 30 minutes later, we ran into Nancy and Tyler again. This time he had assumed his adorable three-year-old self. Relieved, we sat down with him instead of dashing off. Tyler was thrilled and regaled us with stories about his day. His decision to assume a non-bird form was rewarded by our attention and praise. I never saw him as a bird again. Even at age three, it was clear that Tyler was trying on different ways of being and gaining important information about what worked and what didn't by evaluating social rewards and consequences. The bird was an interesting and, fortunately, a brief experiment.

While the responses of neighbors are useful and informative, many of the fundamental stories that we create about our identities were shaped by the perceptions of parents, teachers, and significant others; the more consistent the feedback, the more indelible the story. As we move through adolescence and into adulthood, these personal narratives are interwoven into the fabric of who we are and how we inhabit the world. They also feed forward into the types of experiences and relationships that we seek, and either confirm or refute our beliefs and expectations. More often than not, we seek out information and gravitate to environments and situations that reinforce our personal narratives – a phenomenon referred to as a confirmation bias (Plous 1993).

When I was in grade school my older brother was dubbed the math genius in the family. He was the student who got all As in math without opening a book and received a great deal of recognition. I realized very early on that despite my interest in math, he was the designated genius, which, by default, made me the "non-genius." Over time that identity became part of my personal story. It not only shaped my behavior, but it also had significant bearing on the academic and career choices that I made early in my adult life.

By the time I reached high school, I didn't like math or take advanced level courses because I was "bad " at it. Over time, this "bad at math" story became a limiting belief that steered me away from pursuing a career in science. It was only through my over-whelming desire to pursue a major in psychology and the support of a wonderful math teacher that I eventually discovered that I was quite adept at math. Through practice and perseverance I debunked the myth and rewrote the story. Even so, the original "bad at math" myth still takes hold when I feel challenged by a difficult mathematical dilemma. In other words, stress triggers these stories even when we believe that we've rewritten them. It can almost feel as though they are etched in stone. Even after we erase and replace them, they can still rise to the surface, particularly when we are feeling fearful, overwhelmed, or anxious.

It should be emphasized that not all narratives are negative or harmful and they are certainly not intractable. We live out stories one way or another, some limiting and some empowering. Psychologists Geoffrey Cohen and David Sherman (2014) speak of a mindset in which individuals view themselves as strong, capable, resilient and able to overcome challenge – what they call a narrative of personal adequacy. In a review of the impact of self-affirmation on behavior, they find that positive self-affirmations can and do positively impact health and relationship outcomes, sometimes for months and even years. Conversely, negative narratives can lead to devastating long-term consequences and self-fulfilling prophecies.

In sum, self-narratives ("I am smart," "I am pretty," "I am unlovable," "I fail at relation-ships") are often the central plots to our story lines. We often find ourselves living them out over and over again. We choose experiences that confirm our beliefs, selecting relationships, careers, and situations that affirm these expectations. Our self-narratives can determine how we relate to others and influence the stories we tell ourselves about the people in our lives and how they interact with us. Or, to paraphrase the words of psychologist Abraham Maslow, "if the only tool you have is a hammer, everything looks like a nail" (Maslow 1966). The more you hold to a particular belief, the greater power it wields over you.

Relationships and Learning Histories

Personal stories do not develop in isolation. They are shaped by years of social interac-tion – some positive, some negative. Humans tend to remember painful events more than pleasant ones (Bisby et al. 2016; Vaish, Grossman, & Woodward 2008; Taylor 1991). We are often more likely to recall a critical comment made by a friend than a positive remark – a phenomenon referred to as negativity bias. Research confirms that negative events are usually more salient and remembered and recalled more accurately and in greater detail than positive events. Human language provides an excellent reflection of this. Studies of Western adults find that we have more complex and elaborate language to describe negative emotions and experiences than positive ones.

Negative experiences need not be traumatic to be impactful, but we tend to remember them in remarkable detail and recall them more readily than positive events (see review by Öhman & Mineka 2001). This is particularly true when those emotionally charged incidents occur in the context of a relationship (Fiske 1980; Vaish, Grossman, & Woodward 2008). Imagine a day like any other. You're having what seems to be a perfectly good conversation with your spouse, a friend, a co-worker, or someone you've just met. One minute everything is flowing along smoothly then, in an instant, everything shifts but you're not sure why. You find yourself fumbling to justify, apologize, attack, defend, or back pedal, but no matter how hard you try to right yourself, you've lost your footing and you're going down fast. It can feel remarkably similar to tripping and falling in slow motion. One minute your feet are firmly planted on the ground and the next you've landed flat on your back.

It reminds me of a scene from the comic strip *Peanuts*. In the cartoon, Lucy, the sister of protagonist Charlie Brown's best friend, Linus, repeatedly holds a football for Charlie Brown to kick. She is anything but a kind or compassionate place kicker. For years, she has yanked the football away just as Charlie Brown winds up to kick it, sending him airborne before he slams onto his back. If Charlie Brown just tripped and fell of his own accord he'd probably be embarrassed. But Lucy has pulled the ball out from under him hundreds of times. At this point he's probably not only feeling embarrassed, but hurt, angry, betrayed, and thoroughly fed up. It's one thing to fall on your own, and a very different thing when someone tricks you. In the latter case, we are dealing not only with our own embarrassment, but also the overlay of failing to meet up to our own expectations in the presence of others.

Each of us has a unique learning history shaped by years of social engagement (Bandura 1977; Bandura & Walters 1963). These histories are initially formed in our early childhood relationships with close others. As we develop, we begin to create stories that reflect our identity and vice versa. These often include descriptors from family and close others – "she's smart," "he's a gifted athlete," "she's lazy," "he doesn't get along with others" – and take them to heart. We recite these phrases like mantras until we believe them. Like a stream of water running across the earth, these stories form grooves in our minds that deepen and spread until what was once a story becomes a raging river of rumination.

Why Stories Matter

Why are these stories and personal narratives so important? First, by the time we reach adulthood, these stories and identities are wired into our brains after years of rehearsal. This means that they are likely to be inflexible and habitual features of our mental landscape. Second, we become attached to their content, and are often no longer able to discriminate that they are, in fact, only stories. Third, these stories often operate outside of immediate conscious awareness unless we are primed to remember them. Because of their strength, habitual nature, and the fact that they are strongly linked to our identity, we are particularly susceptible to living them out when we are stressed, tired, anxious, overwhelmed, or fearful.

Think of it this way. If you've ever learned to ride a bicycle, there is a good chance that that skill has been committed to muscle memory. Imagine that I asked you to get onto a bicycle that was altered so that when you turned the handlebars to the right the bike steered to the left? You have probably become so adept at riding a bike that any challenge to your biomechanical memory would throw your balance off. You may even discover that you can't ride the new bicycle because the muscle memory you've acquired to ride a bike is so overlearned that you literally have no idea what to do (if you're curious to see what this looks like, check out www.sciencealert.com/watch-the-mind-bending-science-behind-the-backwards-bicycle). It works similarly for our personal stories. Once they become habitual, it is a considerable challenge to perceive ourselves or situations differently.

Even though our stories influence our perceptions and reactions, we are not destined to live them out. We are, however, much more likely to rely on them as lenses of perception when chronically stressed, emotionally reactive, or acting on autopilot.

You Are What You Think

In the mid-1990s, I began work at the Family Studies Project in the Department of Psychiatry at the University of California at Los Angeles (UCLA) Medical Center. One of my first assignments was to listen to five-minute speech samples of a mother talking about her child and their relationship and to detect characteristics like positivity, criticism, and negative emotion from these narratives. Listening to these speech samples was like being a fly on the wall inside someone's mind. I was mesmerized. Mothers described their children and their relationships with them with impeccable detail. It was remarkable. Our research showed a direct link between a mother's positive or negative perceptions of her child and their relationship, and the child's mental health status. Children whose mothers were critical or negative tended to have higher rates of depression, and those whose mothers expressed positivity were generally better adjusted (Bullock & Asarnow 1998).

This experience had a tremendous impact on my thinking and my interest in exploring the power of personal stories. I wanted to know whether five minutes of audio-recorded speech could predict how parents and their children interacted, and if these interactions directly impacted child and adolescent adjustment and mental health. As a co-investigator on two large, longitudinal, parenting intervention trials, I spent the next decade working with a team that collected several thousand caregiver, youth, adolescent, and young adult speech samples. I created a streamlined version of the original coding scheme so that we could examine these speech samples for affect and attitudes quickly and inexpensively, and use them as clinical feedback tools (Bullock & Dishion 2004; Bullock, Schneiger, & Dishion 2005).

The results from our initial study were astounding. Five minutes of audiotaped narrative during which a caregiver described his or her thoughts and feelings about an adolescent and their relationship reliably predicted observed behavior during a family interaction task. Specifically, caregivers who made one or more critical remarks during the five-minute sample were more likely to be coercive, critical, angry or irritable, and engage in conflict with the teen during a video-recorded family interaction than those who did not make critical remarks. Conversely, caregivers who made positive remarks were more likely to respond to and acknowledge their adolescent and make helpful suggestions, and far less likely to respond with coercion, criticism, anger, irritability or engage in conflict. What's more, caregiver criticism and negativity were significantly associated with adolescent antisocial behavior, whereas positivity served as a protective factor against adolescent lying, stealing, vandalism, aggression, weapon carrying, and other antisocial acts (Bullock & Dishion 2007). This also proved to be the case when looking at the effects of caregiver attitudes on observed interactions with toddlers, and when assessing these children's long-term outcomes (Bullock, Dishion, Gardner, & Shaw 2005; Smith et al. 2013).

The evidence for the link between caregiver attitudes, which we referred to as "relational schemas," observed behavior, and developmental outcomes has, and continues to be, replicated in studies around the world (Pasalich et al. 2011; Waller et al. 2012). Researchers are consistently identifying a link between relational schemas – personal stories that we hold about others – and observed behavior and long-term outcomes. Perhaps the biggest surprise that I witnessed in my own work was that most parents were only vaguely aware of how their attitudes were reflected in their interactions with their children, and how they impacted their children's long-term adjustment. These speech samples became powerful tools in our clinical work with families to cultivate their awareness and to provide motivation for change.

Once you begin to pay attention to your mental chatter, and the stories you tell, you may notice that they may seem endless. It is how the mind works – one incessant stream of commentary. Michael A. Singer, author, essayist, and renowned contemplative educator, suggests that paying attention to this voice is an essential step in liberating ourselves from it. "The best way to free yourself from this incessant chatter is to step back and view it objectively. Just appear like someone there is talking to you. Don't think about it; just notice it," he suggests (Singer 2007, p. 5). But this is easier said than done, particularly when we're stressed, tired, and overtaxed. That's because this voice is very responsive to stress. The more anxious, fearful, and pressured we feel, the louder and more persistent the voice becomes. It's the equivalent of having a hungry toddler in the candy aisle in the grocery store rattling around in your brain. The more you deny it, the more it protests until it gets your attention one way or the other.

Research shows us that we not only have the capacity to pay attention to and stop the chatter of our stories, but we can also reduce our stress, rewire our brains, and reinvent our relationships by responding to them differently (Chan & Woollacott 2007; Hofmann et al. 2010; Moore & Malinowsky 2009). As you will see in the next chapter, this is one of the hallmarks of mindfulness – gently learning to observe and attend to our bodies, minds, and experiences nonjudgmentally. But to make that happen, we first need to learn more about the stories we tell.

EXERCISE
Identifying Your Personal Story

Take a few moments to write down your personal (or organizational) story. You may use simple descriptive phrases like, "I am tough," "I take care of others before myself," or "I am good at math."

You may also choose to write down experiences, family beliefs or other influences that helped to shape how you view yourself now. Once you have listed your beliefs about yourself and identified a few of your stories, look at each one and ask yourself the following questions:

1. Where did this story come from?

2. Is this my story or someone else's?

3. Is this story true of me now?

4. Is this story contributing to or undermining my happiness?

5. Do I choose to continue to live this story or is it time to write a new one?

Collective Stories of Organizations and Systems

Although we often think of stories as the narratives of individuals, they also serve an important function for groups and systems. Group narratives occur in the form of historical stories, mission statements and operational manuals that are created to define goals and objectives and create a shared purpose. They also may be used to delineate organizational culture, socialize new members, generate organizational commitment, and may even function as a form of social control. Similar to our personal stories, these narratives influence attitudes and behavior (Manstead & Fischer 2001).

A mission statement is one example of a narrative designed to articulate a story, or a set of expectations that is intended to be aligned with an organization's goals. Group and organizational harmony occurs when the behaviors of individuals are synchronous with this story. Conversely, organizational dysfunction arises when this narrative is inconsistent with reality. For example, an organization may profess a mission of creating peace and harmony but treat employees with disrespect, or use fear and coercion as management strategies. In this case, there are two organizational narratives – the ideal and the real. The ideal is reflected in the organization's social identity, while the real manifests in narratives of employee dissatisfaction, which can affect job performance, health, and employee relationships.

While a thorough treatment of the role and function of organizational narratives is beyond the scope of this book, it is important to note that the mindsets of groups, organizations, and systems are just as powerful in shaping behavior as personal narratives. These heuristics provide the scaffolding for community cooperation and cohesion. They can also lead to socio-political unrest, divisiveness, partisanship, discrimination, and institutionalized oppression. As such, these stories represent the conscious and unconscious mental events that continuously narrate an organization's experience.

5 | Mindfulness and the Mind

One of the best pieces of advice I ever got was from a horse master. He told me to go slow to go fast. I think that applies to everything in life. We live as though there aren't enough hours in the day but if we do each thing calmly and carefully, we will get it done quicker and with much less stress.

Viggo Mortensen

Mindfulness generally refers to a "quality of consciousness" (Brown & Ryan 2003). Emerging research shows that mindfulness-oriented practices may enhance our wellbeing by grounding our minds and bodies in the present moment, allowing us to examine carefully the thoughts, feelings, sensations, and beliefs that influence our experience (Davis & Hayes 2011; Kabat-Zinn 1990). A state of mindfulness creates discriminant awareness, a space to consider alternative explanations, strategies, and responses to life's circumstances rather than reacting mindlessly. This capacity can be particularly beneficial when we are negotiating difficult or stressful terrain in our relationships.

I believe that mindfulness is inherently relational. Whether in our relationship with ourself or with others, the ability to exercise focused attention, awareness, nonjudgment, and acceptance can enable us to be more compassionate, empathic, and graceful. It can also help us to navigate the various thoughts, feelings, stories, and ways of being that we encounter. A mindful disposition can enable us to be more facile in dealing with the continuous nature of change in our lives and relationships, and to manage the stress that arises as we deal with uncertainty.

In his book, *Full Catastrophe Living: Using the Wisdom of Your Body and Mind to Face Stress, Pain and Illness* (1990), Jon Kabat-Zinn eloquently addresses this relationship between mindfulness and stress. He writes, "The ultimate effect on our health of the total psychological stress we experience depends in large measure on how we come to perceive change itself, in all its various forms, and how skillful we are in adapting to continual change while maintaining our own inner balance and sense of coherence. This, in turn, depends on the meaning we attribute to events, on our beliefs about life and ourselves, and particularly on how much awareness we can bring to our usually mindless and autonomic reactions when our 'buttons' are pushed. It is here, in our mind–body reactions to the occurrences in our lives that we find stressful, that mindfulness most needs to be applied and where its power to transform the quality of our lives can best be put to work" (p. 247).

Mindfulness Research

Although the word "mind" is emphasized in the word mindfulness, mindfulness represents a holistic state, or disposition that includes the mind and body. This may be one reason why contemplative scientists find that mindfulness-oriented practices yield both physical and psychological benefits.

Emerging research shows that mindfulness practices like meditation and yoga may help to reduce the impact of stress-related conditions, ameliorate depressive relapse, lessen depression and anxiety, alleviate pain, improve quality of life, attenuate HIV progression, and increase emotion regulation and subjective well-being (e.g. Baer 2003; Brown, Ryan, & Crewsell 2007; Cherkin et al. 2016; Chisea & Serretti 2009; Creswell et al. 2016; Davis & Hayes 2011; Goyal et al. 2014; Grossman et al. 2004; Khoury et al. 2013; Khoury et al. 2015; Pascoe & Bauer 2015). A large body of evidence also documents the efficacy of mindfulness-based psychotherapeutic interventions in the treatment of depression (Hofmann et al. 2010; Segal et al. 2010; Teasdale et al. 2000), anxiety (Goldin & Gross 2010; Hofmann et al. 2010), eating disorders (Tapper et al. 2009); and chronic pain (Grossman et al. 2007). This may be due, in part, to positive changes in autonomic nervous system (ANS) functioning, including the regulation of heart rate and respiration (Goyal et al. 2014; Streeter et al. 2010, 2012; Telles et al. 2013), as well as changes in brain regions associated with attention, self-regulation, self-control, focused problem-solving, adaptive behavioral coping, interoception, in addition to enhanced memory, reduced emotional interference, and increased cognitive efficiency (Lazar et al. 2005; Gard et al. 2014; Vago & Silbersweig 2012; see Boccia, Piccardi, & Guariglia 2015 for a review). Focused attention meditation, an effortful strategy that requires fixation on a selected object or stimulus, has also been associated with positive psychological outcomes including the recognition of feelings, clarity of thought, positive emotions and well-being, and the ability to control anger.

Meditation and Brain-Related Change

During the past several decades, contemplative neuroscientists have explored how mindfulness practices like meditation may alter brain structure and connectivity and enhance mental function (e.g. Brewer et al. 2011; Creswell et al. 2016; Hölzel et al. 2010, 2011a; Jha, Krompinger, & Baine 2007; Lazar et al. 2005; Tang, Hölzel, & Posner 2015). The brain is composed of neurons (brain cells) and networks (neural connections). The more often we perform a task, the stronger the connections between neurons become. It's sort of like exercising your bicep. The muscle grows bigger and stronger with repeated use. Unlike your muscles, however, networks in the brain are capable not only of increasing in size, but also of changing function depending on how they're used. You've probably heard the expression, "Neurons that fire together wire together" (Shatz 1992). That's a simple way of saying that the efficiency and strength of neural connectivity depends on our behavior. Advances in neuroscience show that we can change neuronal volume and alter the connections that regulate our thoughts, feelings, and behavior in the very same way that we enlarge a muscle – through consistent, repetitive exercise. Frequently employed brain regions show greater cell density, and increased connectivity and efficiency, with consistent use (Simpkins & Simpkins 2013). This applies to both positive and negative thoughts, feelings, and behavior.

Over the past decade, neuroscientists have used brain-imaging techniques like EEG (Davidson et al. 2003), and fMRI (Farb et al. 2010; Lazar et al. 2005; Lutz et al. 2008) to examine how the brain changes when people meditate. They've discovered that experienced meditators show increased volume and activation in their prefrontal cortex (PFC), a region largely responsible for judgment, decision-making, and planning (Lazar et al. 2005). Increased activation of the PFC is linked to prosocial behavior such as empathy, compassion, and kindness. The PFC is important because it can be very susceptible to stress exposure (Arnstein 1999, 2009). Even mildly acute uncontrollable stress can lead to a dramatic decline in prefrontal cognitive abilities, and prolonged stress can result in alterations to the PFC's neural pathways. As such, enhancing PFC volume and activation may serve to buffer the effects of stress and increase cognitive capacities essential for effective communication.

Meditation practice is also related to changes in the anterior cingulate cortex (ACC) and mid-cingulate cortex (MCC). Collectively, the ACC and MCC are associated with self-regulation – the capacity to purposefully direct attention, control impulses, behave thoughtfully and intentionally, and engage in focused problem-solving and adaptive behavioral responses under challenging conditions. People with damage to the ACC tend to be aggressive, impulsive, and rigid in their thinking and persist in using ineffective problem-solving strategies even when they don't work.

A 2014 systematic review and meta-analysis of published studies of neuroimaging of meditation practitioners found that meditators showed differential activation in the ACC and MCC (Fox et al. 2014). Specifically, meditators developed increased ACC and MCC functionality, which may augment self-regulation, attention, and awareness of personal stories. These cognitive and behavioral capacities are particularly important in relationships, as they allow for careful listening, receptivity to other's opinions, and the ability to generate thoughtful responses.

Regular meditation practice is linked to improved learning, memory, and increased self-awareness. A study of 16 adults following an eight-week mindfulness-based stress reduction (MBSR) course demonstrated increases in gray matter in the brain regions associated with perspective-taking, emotion regulation, learning, memory, and self-referential processing. Participants also reported feeling less stress (Hölzel et al. 2011a).

Neuroscientific research also finds that meditation may relate to changes in the limbic system – the region of the brain that processes emotion (Hölzel et al. 2010; Desbordes et al. 2012). As we reviewed in Chapter 2, the limbic system includes the amygdala, a structure that is particularly susceptible to stress. Stress-induced changes to the amygdala are thought to be associated with long-term deficits in cognitive performance, increased emotional – reactivity, as well as pathological levels of anxiety.

Early studies point to changes in amygdalar function and volume following meditation training. For instance, one study found that as little at eight weeks of mindful attention training or cognitively-based compassion training resulted in decreases in right amygdala activation (Desbordes et al. 2012). In a longitudinal MRI study investigating the association between changes in perceived stress and changes in amygdala gray matter density, participants reported significantly less perceived stress following eight weeks of mindfulness-based stress reduction training. What's more, changes in perceived stress correlated significantly with decreases in right basolateral amygdala gray matter density. The more perceived stress was reduced, the less gray matter density in the right amygdala (Hölzel et al. 2010). This implies that regular meditation may stimulate neuroplasticity, which may directly safeguard against impact of stress, and potentially increase emotional resilience.

The default mode network (DMN), which is sometimes referred to as the "monkey mind," is another structure that appears to be impacted by meditation practice (Brewer et al. 2011; Garrison et al. 2015; Jang et al. 2011; Tomasino et al. 2013). The DMN is represented by a number of highly interconnected structures including the posterior cingulate cortex (PCC), dorsolateral (dlPFC), and medial prefrontal cortex (mPFC), angular gyrus, precuneus, and hippocampus. The DMN is associated with three primary functions: self-referencing, thinking about others, and recalling the past and anticipating future events. Research shows that this network is vulnerable to fear and stress and may play an important role in depression, chronic pain, schizophrenia, autism spectrum disorders, and Alzheimer's disease (Buckner, Andrews-Hanna, & Schacter 2008).

The DMN is increasingly gaining attention because of its role in social information processing. A highly active DMN may be a marker of perseverative rumination, or personal stories running amok. In one study, Judson Brewer, Director of Research at the Center for Mindfulness at the University of Massachusetts, found that the DMN was "relatively deactivated" in experienced meditators, suggesting that meditation may help to reduce mind wandering and possibly rumination (Brewer et al. 2011).

J. David Creswell and colleagues at Carnegie Mellon University examined the relationship between the DMN and physiological markers of stress in a highly stressed population of job seeking adults (Creswell et al. 2009). Thirty-five participants were randomly assigned to an intensive, three-day, residential mindfulness meditation retreat or a relaxation retreat. Resting brain scans and blood tests were taken immediately before and after the intervention, and blood was again drawn at a four-month follow-up. Post-intervention scans showed increased resting state functional connectivity of regions of the DMN associated with attention and executive control (dlPFC) in the meditation group only. The meditation group also had reduced interleukin-6 levels, which suggests an attenuated inflammatory response. These findings show that meditation may enhance executive control and stress regulation, in addition to affecting stress-related health indicators like inflammation. Indeed, a meta-analysis of neuroimaging studies that included data from 24 experiments found consistent evidence that meditation is associated with changes in executive attention function, including functional alterations in the default mode network (Tomasino et al. 2013).

Yoga researchers have also detected neurobiological changes following regular yoga practice (Streeter et al. 2010, 2012). In a 2010 study, Dr. Chris Streeter, Associate Professor of Psychiatry at Boston University School of Medicine and Boston Medical Center, and her colleagues randomly assigned adult participants to either a yoga intervention or an active walking group. Both yoga and walking group members participated in three, 60-minute sessions per week for 12 weeks. Greater improvements in self-reported mood and anxiety ratings were found in the yoga group compared to the walking group at the end of the study. Yoga participants also showed a positive correlation between improved mood and decreased anxiety and increased thalamic GABA levels (Streeter et al. 2010). GABA, or gamma-amniobutyric acid, is a primary inhibitory neurotransmitter in the brain, whose primary function is relaxation. Depleted GABA activity is linked to depression, anxiety, panic disorder, aggressive and antisocial behavior, substance abuse, epilepsy, and chronic pain. These metabolic changes in the brain, associated with enhanced mood and reduced anxiety, may occur following regular yoga practice. Streeter believes that changes in GABA levels may be related to activity in the parasympathetic nervous system (PNS), which increases GABA activation in brain structures responsible for stress reactivity, emotion regulation, and threat perception.

One of the most promising and impactful benefits of mindfulness practice may be in its ability to reduce stress. According to the World Health Organization, worker stress costs American businesses approximately $300 billion per year, predominantly in the form of higher healthcare costs, employee absence, and reduced productivity. A review of 25 randomized controlled trials examined the published evidence of the effects of breathing exercises, yoga, meditation, and other mindfulness practices (or their combination) on the sympathetic nervous system and hypothalamic pituitary adrenal (HPA)-axis – both of which are well-known indicators of stress (Pascoe & Bauer 2015). It included studies that measured structural and/or functional brain regions associated with stress and mood regulation, as well as other physiological indicators like heart rate, blood pressure, and cortisol levels. In this review, mindfulness practices were found to be associated with improved SNS and HPA-axis regulation, as well as decreased symptoms of anxiety and depression across a diverse range of participants. Similarly, a review and meta-analysis of seven controlled and randomized controlled trials, in which MBSR was compared to other forms of treatment in the relief of stress and stress-related symptoms in healthy individuals, found that MBSR participants reported reduced stress and fewer symptoms of ruminative thinking and anxiety, as well as increased self-compassion and empathy (Chisea & Seretti 2009).

Mindfulness and Relationship Satisfaction

Contemplative science has focused predominantly on individual differences that vary as a function of state or dispositional mindfulness. There is an increasing recognition among scientists that mindfulness is also inherently relational, with capacities such as focused attention, awareness, nonjudgment, and experiential acceptance being hallmarks of good interpersonal engagement. Indeed, psychotherapeutic approaches, such as Acceptance and Commitment Therapy (ACT; Hayes, Strosahl & Wilson 1999), Dialectical Behavioral Therapy (DBT; Linehan 1993), Integrative Behavioral Couples Therapy (IBCT; Jacobson & Christensen 1996), and Mindfulness–Based Cognitive Therapy (MBCT; Segal et al. 2004), have long recognized the impact of mindfulness for psychological and relational health, integrating mindfulness skills, practices, and philosophy into cognitive, behavioral, and behavior analytic therapies for decades.

An emergent body of research shows that mindfulness positively impacts social connectedness, perspective taking, and social skills, is linked to greater acceptance and fewer avoidant behaviors, and is associated with reduced negative reactivity during interpersonal conflict in romantic relationships (Barnes et al. 2007; Burpee & Langer 2005; Carson et al. 2004; Gambrel & Piercy 2014a, 2014b; Jacobson & Christensen 1996). In addition, those identified as mindful tend to experience enhanced relationship quality and satisfaction (Barnes et al. 2007; Kozlowski 2013).

A number of interventions designed to cultivate mindfulness have also been found to enhance relationship satisfaction. A 2013 literature review and synopsis of studies examining the association between an individual's level of mindfulness and relationship satisfaction reported that higher levels of both dispositional mindfulness and skills learned through mindfulness training are related to higher relationship satisfaction (Kozlowski 2013). More recently, a statistical meta-analysis of 12 studies (published research and unpublished doctoral dissertations) conducted between 2005 and 2014 revealed small to moderate, statistically significant effects linking higher levels of mindfulness with greater relationship satisfaction (McGill, Adler-Baeder, & Rodriguez 2016). This association may be due to the increased ability of mindful individuals to manage stress, regulate their emotions, respond to others empathically, and communicate effectively.

As the popularity of mindfulness for relationship enhancement grows, so do related educational programs. Carson and colleagues studied the effectiveness of a mindfulness-based relationship education program on marital quality. They found that, in a sample of nondistressed couples, both mindfulness and relationship satisfaction increased following participation in the program (Carson et al. 2004). Gambrel and Piercy (2014b) also found that mindfulness-oriented education increased mindfulness and relationship satisfaction in a sample of expectant parents. Together, these data point to mindfulness training as benefitting both individuals and those with whom they share relationships.

Mindfulness and Narrative – Separating Fact from Fiction

Mindfulness strategies that reduce stress and increase positivity focus on unlearning habitual responses and considering alternate thoughts or behaviors. Although we have yet to learn the specific mechanisms needed to accomplish this, several interesting studies suggest that practices like meditation work the "mental muscles" associated with our ability to maintain focused attention and/or inhibit automatic or habitual responses (Hölzel et al. 2011b; Lutz et al. 2009; Moore et al. 2012; Wenk-Sormaz 2005).

Our ability to manage our thoughts by inhibiting one response and doing something else is referred to as directed attention. When we possess the capacity for directed attention, we can voluntarily impede certain automatic cognitive processes, (for example, the stories we tell about others and ourselves) and direct our thoughts elsewhere. This doesn't mean that we aren't aware of our stories. Rather, by inhibiting our habitual reliance on them, we gain the capacity to question them or divert our attention away from them toward thoughts, feelings, or behaviors that may be more healthy or adaptive.

Several studies support the proposition that mindfulness practices like meditation enhance directed attention. In one such study, 40 adults with no prior history of meditation practice were randomly assigned to either a meditation group or a wait list control group. Meditation group participants received three hours of mindfulness meditation training. Of the 28 participants who were compared in the final analysis, meditators were found to have greater improvements in attentional resources and cognitive efficiency than controls (Moore et al. 2012). Specifically, meditators successfully completed more items on the Stroop task, and made fewer errors than non-meditators. Their enhanced performance was directly correlated with higher mindfulness scores. Other studies find that meditators demonstrate less cognitive interference than non-meditators. While far from conclusive, this introduces the possibility that mindfulness practices that focus attention may be useful in enabling us to pay attention to, and discriminate between, our personal narratives and our present experience, allowing for greater cognitive flexibility and more present-focused and adaptive responding.

Dispelling Mindfulness Myths

Although often attributed to Buddhism, most major faith and wisdom traditions have long made use of practices designed to cultivate a mindful disposition or state. In recent history, mindfulness has been secularized by mainstream society and its emphasis, for some, has shifted from a practice of transcendence to a means for decreasing stress, increasing attention, awareness, and personal success. This has led to criticism of mindfulness both epistemologically and empirically (e.g. Sharf 2015). In regards to the latter, the emerging field of contemplative science continues to grapple with a lack of operational and conceptual agreement, methodological concerns, and considerable heterogeneity of practices/interventions and measurement strategies (Vago & Silbersweig 2012). In spite of this, the empirical literature broadly supports the premise that a mindful state or disposition may be beneficial for many individuals, enabling them to be aware of the ways in which their personal stories and habitual behaviors cause illness and suffering (Boccia, Piccardi, & Guariglia 2015; Khoury et al. 2013, 2015).

The increased popularity and secularization of mindfulness has also kindled myths and controversy. Survey claims of the effects of mindfulness and meditation range from completely rewiring your brain to thwarting aging or attaining professional or athletic success. Search Google for the "effects of mindfulness" and you will find definitive claims that mindfulness "reform[s] the structure of the brain," that "thousands of peer-reviewed scientific papers prove that mindfulness enhances mental and physical wellbeing and reduces chronic pain, " and "mindfulness is at least as good as drugs or counseling for the treatment of clinical-level depression." That is only the beginning.

Mindfulness is now a billion dollar industry. Sitting meditation has become a staple in an impressive array of corporations (Google, eBay, Apple, Aetna, General Mills, General Motors, IBM, Patagonia, and Goldman Sachs for starters), business schools (Harvard University, Georgetown University, New York University), title-winning professional sports franchises (Chicago Bulls and Seattle Seahawks), not to mention the United States military (M-fit). Search "meditation" on Amazon.com and you will find nearly 400,000 hits for everything from books, CDs, meditation timers, cushions, incense, prayer beads, and Buddha statues, to headbands that claim to let "you hear what's happening in your brain while you meditate." That's remarkable, if not paradoxical. If a function of meditation is to cultivate awareness, why would you need a device to inform you when you've arrived?

Part of the reason for this phenomenon is that mindfulness sells. And the more it is presented as a quick fix to our ills, the more it will continue to do so. But mindfulness is far from a quick fix. It requires time, effort, and a willingness to experience not only relaxed states, but difficult and painful ones as well. That may be one reason why many people choose not to meditate in spite of myriad programs and meditation groups offered in boardrooms, retreat centers, strip malls, schools, hospitals, and beyond.

Why Don't People Meditate?

According to a recent National Health Statistics Report, the overwhelming majority of Americans, approximately 92%, do not meditate (Clarke et al. 2015). In reading this statistic, I became curious as to why. I began by examining the research and media accounts and commentaries about the negative effects of mindfulness practice, discovering a lesser known but as equally powerful movement toward skepticism. Intrigued by these results, I conducted informal research, asking friends, colleagues, students, workshop participants, and others about their feelings on meditation and mindfulness. What I discovered included an emerging backlash against the mindfulness movement, not to mention some fascinating perceptions about mindfulness and meditation.

As popular as mindfulness has become, many continue to resist claims that it is a one-size-fits-all "magic pill." Indeed, the proliferation of hype about the benefits of mindfulness has ignited considerable skepticism. Buddhist teacher-scholars Ron Purser and David Loy, authors of the 2013 Huffington Post blog, *Beyond McMindfulness*, fear that mainstream American mindfulness has devolved from a practice to a commodity, becoming nothing more than a commercialized self-help craze. Others, like journalist Mary Sykes Wylie in her 2015 article, *How the Mindfulness Movement Went Mainstream – And the Backlash That Came With It*, contend that mindfulness has been "individualized, monetized, corporatized, therapized, taken over, flattened, and generally co-opted out of all resemblance to its noble origins in an ancient spiritual and moral tradition" (Sykes Wylie 2015).

Even contemplative scientists are calling for greater prudence in reporting the outcomes of mindfulness studies. Catherine Kerr, Assistant Professor of Medicine at Brown University, who directs translational neuroscience for Brown's Contemplative Studies Initiative, has repeatedly called for a tempered approach to communicating research findings. In the May 14, 2014 entry on her personal Facebook page, she posted the article *LOOK: What Meditation Can Do to Your Mind, Body, and Spirit* along with the following comment: "… it's not like any of [the claims of the benefits of mindfulness practice are] grossly inaccurate… it's just that the studies are too cherry-picked and too positive and the piece does not talk about the fact that meditation may not be suitable for all people in all circumstances." She goes on to say, "I think we are all going to need to take responsibility and do something so that the coverage looks slightly more balanced – otherwise, when the inevitably negative studies come, this whole wave will come crashing down on us."

This tendency toward an imbalance of positivity is reflected in recent meta-analysis of 124 published trials of mindfulness-based therapies that found that 88% were reported to be effective. This figure is 1.6 times the anticipated number of positive results based on what would be expected statistically, leading the study's authors to conclude, "the proportion of mindfulness-based therapy trials with statistically significant results may overstate what would occur in practice" (Coronado-Montoya et al. 2016).

That wave may have already started to break. A 2014 review of randomized controlled trials examining the effects of meditation for alleviating psychological distress including pain found only 47 published peer-reviewed articles (Goyal et al. 2014). Even factoring in the two years since this review was conducted, this is very different from the thousands noted above. From a research perspective, these studies represent the emergence of evidence, not a sufficient body of data from which to make definitive assertions. Yet, in spite of this, claims of mindfulness as a cure-all continue to blanket every segment of the media. This raises the suspicion that mindfulness is just another fad and that the supporting research is a house of cards. As Kerr notes in a 2014 interview entitled, "Don't Believe the Hype," published in a 2014 issue of *Tricycle*, "People will lose faith and revert to the other side: mindfulness has no value." Many have.

Clearly, the story around the risks and rewards of mindfulness and meditation practice is far from black and white. Research points to both its benefits as well as its negative effects, particularly for those with existing psychiatric conditions, a history of traumatic experiences, or PTSD. For many, sitting with their thoughts and experiences is foreign, and sometimes hostile, territory. In the 2015 book *The Buddha Pill: Can Meditation Change You?*, psychologists Miguel Farias and Catherine Wilkholm provide a balanced, historical account of the empirical evidence in support of mindfulness education and the pitfalls of the practice (Farias & Wilkholm 2015). Their compelling examination of the emerging research led them to conclude that much is to be learned of both the benefits and the risks of meditation and yoga. They are also clear to point out that mindfulness practices are far from a panacea, and that delusional thinking and dismissal of adverse events and experiences will only serve to diminish the true benefits of these practices.

Media hype and tenuous science aside, there is one compelling reason why people don't practice sitting meditation – most people can't sit still. This first hit me while working on a mindfulness program for first-time, low-income mothers of toddlers. Initially, I began with all of these wonderful ideas of introducing moms to some simple yoga, breath, and meditation practices for relieving stress. But as I developed the program, one image from my earlier clinical work continued to haunt me – a two-year-old having a meltdown in the grocery store line. You know, the toddler turned terrorist grabbing for candy and scratching, kicking, and screaming, "I WANT IT!" at the top of their lungs. Their mom, flushed, tries desperately to calm her youngster as a sea of disapproving faces look on. Would a meditation practice be of benefit? Would an already busy, harried parent be able to sit still when her stress level was mounting or already off the charts? Perhaps, but the odds are probably low, assuming that she'd been able to find the time to meditate with a toddler at home in the first place.

This got me to wondering if meditation was truly the answer. I began interviewing clients, friends, posting questions on social media, and asking anyone who would respond about their feelings on meditation. By far the number one reason most people took up meditation was to reduce stress. Ironically, the number one reason why people chose not to partake in sitting meditation was also because of high levels of stress. This was followed by an inability to sit still and not having the time.

Nate, an attendee at one of my BREATHE workshops, described his difficulty with sitting meditation this way. "It's like my system is in overdrive. I'm pressing the gas pedal to the floor and I'm not moving. Instead of feeling calm, my engine is revving and I'm bouncing off the walls. I can't let my foot off the gas pedal because I'm exhausted. I'm afraid that the engine won't start again. I feel stuck." Having tried and failed at meditation more than once, Nate concluded that it isn't for him. He arrived at my workshop hoping to find a different path to mindfuless that did not require him to sit still for lengthy periods of time.

What I discovered is that people adopt what works for them. Many non-meditators reported engaging in other activities to gain peace and perspective such as running, yoga, hiking, and walking. Julia, a 65-year-old psychologist, said, "I'm the walking in nature type of meditating person." Allison, a 39-year-old customer service representative, reported, "I use running to ground me. If I'm not able to get in some hard exercise, my mind begins to spin out and I can get wired and anxious. Moving is my meditation." They are not alone. A 2014 report issued by the U.S. Department of Health and Human Services indicates that nearly 50% of American adults 18 years of age or over engage in vigorous aerobic exercise a minimum of 75 minutes per week, or moderate-intensity activity for 2½ hours per week. For them, moving is meditation.

In addition to having a hard time sitting still, many I asked were perplexed by the idea of quieting the mind. There's a good reason for this. As we discovered in Chapter 4, we make sense of the world through language and relate to our experience by way of stories. Our minds are in a continuous state of chatter, and, by and large, we've become habituated to it. Our minds are like a radio playing nonstop in the background; we aren't always aware of the message infiltrating our stream of consciousness, but it is there, particularly when we turn up the volume. Even in our dreams, our minds sift through the residue of the day or a lifetime that we may have insufficiently attended to. Most of us don't even realize that the stories are playing until we sit still long enough to hear them.

Stephen, a 52-year-old auto mechanic, describes his experience with meditation this way. "Some of us don't get it, directly. 'Hmm, I can tell that this is going to be a long five minutes. I am supposed to sit and think. About what? Myself? Why? Contort myself? Ouch. Now I get to think about the pain. What to do when I get done with this? Sure hope no one is staring at me realizing I'm not meditating. OK. Four minutes left. This is just like praying when you sneak peeks at the others who are praying. I'm hungry. Is this what meditation is for, to help you know when you are hungry? It works! Three minutes left… Why do they call Red Vines licorice? Licorice is a flavor, not a color. Two minutes… That car at work sure is driving me nuts. Why do I have this recurring issue? I have changed so many parts, what am I missing? Maybe tonight I will think about it and figure it out… Two minutes… Do dogs meditate? Hmmm. When I get done I need to get mowing the lawn; riding the lawn mower sure lets you relax and think. One minute… My leg is cramping. How often am I supposed to do this? OUCH, OUCH, OUCH! Whew. All done. Now what was the point of this?'"

Stephen is not alone. Most people I interviewed reported that sitting still for any length of time is nearly as painful as a root canal. So, they avoid it. Does this mean that they're missing out on the ultimate experience of mindfuless? Absolutely not, but not everyone agrees.

David Gelles, author of *Mindful Work: How Meditation is Changing Business From the Inside Out* (Gelles 2015), contends that meditation is the *sine qua non* of mindfulness practices. He bases his contention on the emerging literature attesting to the benefits of the practice for everything from increasing gray matter to alleviating irritable bowel syndrome (IBS). However, there are a lot of missing pieces to mindfulness research. We have no idea why the practices work or how. While associating meditation with brain change is interesting, alterations in brain size, structure, and connectivity don't necessarily have a one-to-one relationship to "mindful" behavior. We have but a glimpse of the mechanism through which meditation works to cultivate mindfulness, but don't really know whether a mindful state or disposition is reliably associated with increased socio-emotional intelligence or skillful action. We know nothing about the optimal "dose" of meditation or whether the effects of meditation persist if people practice intermittently or stop meditating altogether.

Perhaps even more importantly, the negative effects of meditation have largely been dismissed, unreported, or ignored until recently. Willoughby Britton, Assistant Professor of Psychiatry and Human Behavior at Brown University Medical School and long-time meditation practitioner, was one of the first researchers to draw attention not only to this issue, but the potential for bias as well. In a 2014 interview, "Meditation Nation," published in *Tricycle*, Britton discussed the potential negative effects of meditation as well as the tendency for contemplative science to endorse its own beliefs. Her research shows that, for some, meditation can lead to psychological crises and severe, long-term impairment. "In the Buddhist community, there are a lot of people who are excited about the scientific findings that support the efficacy of meditation because it seems to be confirming what we already knew," she says. "But that is not the purpose of science – to confirm the dharma. And if that is what people are doing as scientists, they need to seriously step back and look at the ethics of that. To use science to prove your religion or worldview – there is something really wrong with that." Britton recommends less hype and the acknowledgment of the pitfalls of the practice in addition to its benefits – a conversation that has, until recent years, been shoved under the rug and overlooked by mainstream media and proponents of mindfulness meditation.

"People still aren't clear about [what mindfulness is]," says Britton. "What are these different practices? And which practices are best or worst suited to which types of people? When is it skillful to stop meditating and do something else? I think that this is the most logical direction to follow because nothing is good for everyone. Mindfulness is not going to be an exception to that."

Meditation isn't for everyone. As mentioned above, it is also not the only path to mindfulness. Many people turn to yoga, tai chi, and other forms of "moving meditation" to satisfy their need for a contemplative practice. A 2012 National Health Statistics Report suggests that slightly more (10.1%) adults now practice yoga, tai chi, and Qigong than in previous years (Clarke et al. 2015). This is up from 6.7% in 2007. With yoga and meditation combined, roughly 18% of U.S. adults take time out of their busy lives to engage in some form of mindfulness practice. What about the other 82%?

Based on the findings of my informal research, it is likely that many find solace in activities like prayer, music, cooking, gardening, hiking, mountain climbing, art, and various other physical and expressive outlets. We don't really know whether or how their effects parallel formal sitting meditation practice, but the science tells us that they have similar neurophysiological benefits. Does this mean that we should toss out the idea of mindfulness altogether and let people live and let live? I don't have the answer to that question. I do know that, regardless of what activities you pursue, you are likely to be confronted with an inordinate amount of life stress at some point in time, and there is one tool at your disposal that can help to quickly mitigate its effects – the breath.

6 | Personal Responsibility and Social Change

It is not our purpose to become each other; it is to recognize each other, to learn to see the other and honor him for what he is.

Hermann Hesse

Our world is as magnificent and glorious as it is troubled. Roughly one billion of the nearly 7.5 billion of this planet's human inhabitants struggle to subsist. The Earth's climate reflects the cataclysmic consequences of human propagation and consumption. Divisiveness, war, discrimination, oppression, and religious persecution define much of our socio-political landscape. Disease, homelessness, and mental illness are rampant. As we learned in prior chapters, stress can either lead to an expansion of consciousness as we rise to meet the challenges of our age, or turn us toward blame, criticism, contempt, defensiveness, and, in the extreme, violence. Just as we each run the risk of harming others by denying the impact of chronic stress on our wellbeing, human systems and those responsible for running them face the risk of a similar fate. Systems are, after all, made up of people.

We need to shift our mindset to recognize and acknowledge that the needs of the many outweigh the needs of the few. This necessitates taking stock of our thoughts, feelings, behaviors, and lives and becoming aware of how each feeds into our day-to-day experience, and that of others and our planet. It means being aware of the role that stress and the stories we tell play in our experience, and using that knowledge to inform our actions. It requires acknowledging both the good and the shadow sides of our nature and, rather than criticizing or ignoring our imperfections, embracing them and using that subjective reality to initiate personal and social change.

Stress, Social Roles, and Responsibility

As we learned earlier, the stories that we tell have large bearing on the social roles that we assume, and the ways in which we relate to ourselves and the world. Even though they may seem relatively fixed, these stories are also malleable depending on the context in which we find ourselves. This is poignantly illustrated in the novel, *Lord of the Flies*, written by Nobel Prize-winning author William Golding (1962). In the story, a British plane crashes on a desolate island in the Pacific Ocean during a wartime evacuation. The only survivors are preadolescent boys who belonged to one of two groups – ordinary students or a boys' choir. On the island, the boys quickly form two groups – the first consisting of the ordinary students organized by a popular boy named Ralph, and the second consisting of members of the choir led by their student director, Jack.

The book chronicles the boys' descent into savagery as they struggle to subsist. Group identities are formed and ideologies around survival, pleasure, and aggression are established. Some students are persecuted for their differences, leadership is threatened, and they devolve into a pack of brutes, inevitably killing one of the boys and torturing several others. Eventually the boys are rescued, but only once the darkness in their hearts has been revealed. They have come to face what Carl Jung refers to as the shadow – the unknown dark side of human personality that often lies dormant and out of conscious awareness (Jung 1938). It is a lesson for us all. A shadow left unacknowledged can be the most dangerous threat of all.

Psychological research confirms that people are capable of engaging in unspeakable acts, particularly when under extreme duress or while deferring to a perceived authority. A classic social psychology study, conducted in 1963 by Stanley Milgram, a psychologist at Yale University, examined whether a person would follow the instructions of an authority figure, even if those instructions were in direct conflict with his or her beliefs (Milgram 1963). Milgram was motivated by the trial of Adolf Eichmann, a German Nazi lieutenant colonel known for being a key organizer of the holocaust during World War II. In spite of his role in the mass killing of millions, Eichmann's attorneys argued that he was merely following orders. Eichmann himself refused to admit personal responsibility, stating, "I was one of the many horses pulling the wagon and couldn't escape left or right because of the will of the driver."

Milgram recruited men between the ages of 20 and 50 to participate in a study of "learning," telling them that they would be randomly designated as either a "teacher" or a "learner." This randomization was rigged so that participants would always be the teacher and a confederate of Milgram, "Mr. Wallace," would always be the learner. Each participant and Mr. Wallace were led to the Yale Interaction Laboratory where Mr. Wallace was strapped to a sham electric chair and fitted with electrodes. The teacher was then escorted to a separate room with an electric shock generator. Shock values ranged from a low of 15 volts (low) to 450 (severe or potentially lethal) and were clearly marked on each of the 30 switches in the shock generator. The experimenter was positioned behind the teacher to provide instruction.

Mr. Wallace was instructed to memorize a list of word pairs. Once Mr. Wallace had learned the list, the teacher named a word and instructed Mr. Wallace to provide the corresponding correct response from a list of four options. The teacher was instructed to administer an electric shock each time Mr. Wallace made a mistake, and to increase the level of shock incrementally with each subsequent error. What the teacher did not know was that Mr. Wallace was intentionally providing wrong answers so that the teacher was forced to administer a shock. When teachers refused to shock Mr. Wallace, they were given a standardized series of increasingly demonstrative directives by the experimenter ("please continue," "the experiment requires you to continue," "it is absolutely essential that you continue," and "you have no other choice but to continue").

Nearly two-thirds (65%) of participants continued increasing the voltage inflicted on Mr. Wallace up to the maximum 450 volts, despite knowing that they may be causing lethal harm. All of the participants administered up to 300 volts of shock. Milgram achieved similar results in 18 subsequent studies. In his famous 1973 article entitled, "The Perils of Obedience," he concluded that people assume one of two potential behavioral states when responding to social cues: autonomous or agentic. In an autonomous state, people take responsibility for their behavior. In an agentic state, they follow the instructions of an authority figure and abdicate responsibility for their actions. He stated,

"The legal and philosophical aspects of obedience are of enormous import, but they say very little about how most people behave in concrete situations. I set up a simple experiment at Yale University to test how much pain an ordinary citizen would inflict on another person simply because he was ordered to by an experimental scientist. Stark authority was pitted against the subjects' [participants'] strongest moral imperatives against hurting others, and, with the subjects' [participants'] ears ringing with the screams of the victims, authority won more often than not. The extreme willingness of adults to go to almost any lengths on the command of an authority constitutes the chief finding of the study and the fact most urgently demanding explanation" (Milgram 1963, p. 375).

In other words, social pressures can compel us to do almost anything, including modifying the stories that we tell about who we are and the lengths we might go to when experiencing extreme stress.

In 1971, Stanford University psychologist Philip Zimbardo assembled a group of middle-class, male college students screened for having no current psychological problems. He randomly assigned each to be either a "prisoner" or a "prison guard" in what became the infamous Zimbardo Prison Study (Haney, Banks, & Zimbardo 1973). Each of the 10 men selected as prisoners was visited by local police officers and arrested, searched, and handcuffed. Prisoners were then placed in the back of a squad car, driven to the local police station, booked, fingerprinted, and placed in a holding cell where they were blindfolded and later transported to a mock prison in the Stanford University psychology department where they were stripped, deloused, and given a numbered uniform that resembled a dress.

The 11 men who were randomly assigned to guard the prisoners were offered little instruction. They were outfitted in khaki uniforms and given whistles, nightsticks, and mirrored sunglasses. In the days that followed, these seemingly unremarkable students morphed into personalities that reflected their assigned roles. Within hours guards became hostile, sadistic, and aggressive. They assigned prisoners meaningless, demoralizing tasks. Prisoners became increasingly more passive, submissive, and depressed and guards became increasingly more hostile. After 36 hours, one prisoner was removed from the study because of uncontrollable fits of anger, screaming, and crying. Although intended to last two weeks, the study was terminated after six days due to the escalating brutality of the guards and the distress of participants. In later interviews, many of the guards reported that they were acting out a role and did not believe that they were capable of similar behaviors in real life. The researchers concluded that the behavior of participants was driven by the situation, not a reflection of their disposition or character.

The Milgram and Zimbardo studies suggest that, when in certain social situations or under duress, we have the potential to behave in ways that conflict with our personal beliefs, values, and stories. This is particularly true when we feel social pressure to conform to the stories of others.

Stress and Systems

Sociological research shows that leaders, and others within organizations and systems, tend to exhibit the same stress-related behaviors as others when faced with real or perceived danger. When under duress, attention narrows or becomes fixated, information processing is simplified, and thoughts become more rigid (Janis 1982). This can significantly reduce effective decision-making. As we saw with Suzanne, Tal, and Yolanda earlier, we are more likely to become fearful, aggressive, defensive, and to live out our stories when the stresses of our life seem greater than we can handle. In the context of organizations and systems, we may defer decision-making to authority figures. This isn't necessarily advantageous, as leaders are also more likely to draw on pre-existing mindsets, personal narratives, rigid thinking, and habitual strategies when in states of chronic stress.

Peter Senge, systems scientist, founder of the Society for Organizational Learning and author of *The Fifth Discipline: The Art & Practice of the Learning Organization*, describes decision-making using organizational psychologist Chris Argyris' Ladder of Inference model (Senge 2006; Figure 6.1). The Ladder of Inference proposes that leaders adopt behaviors that reflect or confirm their personal narratives, and that they create contexts and circumstances that verify or maintain their personal stories. Similarly

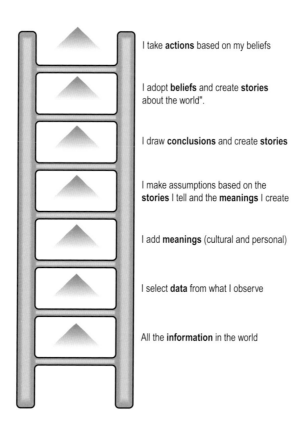

I take **actions** based on my beliefs

I adopt **beliefs** and create **stories** about the world".

I draw **conclusions** and create **stories**

I make assumptions based on the **stories** I tell and the **meanings** I create

I add **meanings** (cultural and personal)

I select **data** from what I observe

All the **information** in the world

Figure 6.1
Ladder of inference

to how Yolanda suffered from the imposter effect and chose to micromanage her staff, or how Suzanne responded to others fearfully when believing she was about to lose her job, leaders and workers use existing schemas to interpret and respond to their organizational milieu. This means that, particularly when in states of chronic stress, they are apt to filter out observations that are inconsistent with their ideologies and attend to information that concurs with their beliefs.

Under these circumstances, positive results are seen as confirmation of individuals' biases, reinforcing that their perceptions or decisions were "right." This increases the likelihood that similar strategies and attitudes will be adopted in the future. Conversely, negative results may be dismissed or ignored because they don't conform to individuals' stories. In sum, individuals within organizations adopt norms, ideologies, mission statements, and other tools that solidify their belief systems. The more these assumptions are left untested, and to the extent that they are reinforced, the more concretized they become. This is advantageous in healthy work environments in which individuals and leaders engage in open, respective communication, or in which evaluation of performance and outcome is handled fairly. It can, however, be detrimental in circumstances in which workers feel marginalized, or where leaders or organizations fail to examine the impact of their behavior.

Whether as individuals or in systems, the more we believe that our stories reflect the "truth," and our assumptions remain untested, the more rigid in our thinking and behavior we are likely to become. This can lead to polarization and intolerance of those whose beliefs or behaviors are dissimilar from our own. In-group/out-group biases are powerful examples of this rigidity. In the early twentieth century, sociologist William Sumner argued that humans tend to categorize themselves and others into in-groups ("we-groups") and out-groups ("others-groups"). This is particularly the case under conditions in which individuals believe that they are struggling for their existence (Sumner 1906). Sumner writes,

"The insiders in a we-group are in a relation of peace, order, law, government, and industry, to each other. Their relation to all outsiders, or others-groups, is one of war and plunder... Sentiments are produced to correspond. Loyalty to the group, sacrifice for it, hatred and contempt for outsiders, brotherhood within, warlikeness without – all grow together, common products of the same situation" (Sumner 1906, p. 12).

Although in-group connections often are formed intentionally and out of shared purpose, these groups can also be formed chaotically, rapidly, and in response to high levels of fear or threat. They are often the underlying impetus behind violence, war, and misguided social policies that exclude, discriminate, or ostracize dissimilar others.

In-group/out-group biases are reflections of personal stories and mindsets. We define our social identity and respond to others based on perceived similarities and differences. These narratives are, by default, dualistic. If I am a resident of city 'x' then I am not a resident of city 'y'. Similarly, if I am female, I am not male. If I am of mixed race, I am not exclusively Hispanic, African American, or Inuit. We use classifications on an ongoing basis to evaluate threat, safety, attraction, likability, and so on. While we may believe we are in touch with our attitudes, the automatic assumptions that we make are often implicit and unconscious, particularly when we are in a state of chronic stress.

Physical appearance is usually the first line of information that we attend to (Devine 1989). We make immediate associations and judgments based on visual cues like dress, skin color, posture, and other nonverbal information (facial expression, pupil dilation, body size, health and disability cues, gender, attractiveness, etc.). We are inclined to assign more positive attributes to those whom we perceive to be similar to us and vice versa. It's important to know that these social constructions are key features of our personal stories.

The term "othering" refers to any action by which we classify a person or group as not one of us. Like in-group and out-group biases, othering is thought to have an evolutionary function (Dervin 2012). In early human history, it was essential to have an allegiance to one's kin or social group to survive. The more resources that could be pooled to hunt, gather, protect, nurture, and procreate, the more likely the tribe was to survive. As human civilizations expanded, these social constructions gained in complexity. In addition to age, gender, relationship, physical similarity, race, and social status factors such as religious affiliation, dress, political affiliation, wealth, power, and the size of one's army, became important considerations in establishing connectedness to others to maximize personal gain and safety and minimize danger and social isolation.

Prejudice and discrimination are outward manifestations of individual, neural, and socially constructed narratives about dissimilar others (Reynolds et al. 2014). These stories are largely shaped by social groups, learned experience, and context. Experiments have revealed how quickly and readily we can change these classifications as well as our behavior toward dissimilar others. The Brown Eyes, Blue Eyes Study was conducted by Jane Elliott, a third and fourth grade elementary school teacher in a small town in Iowa in the 1960s (Peters 1971). Inspired by the death of Martin Luther King and wanting to teach her students about racial discrimination, Elliott decided to conduct a brief experiment. One day she told her students that research suggested that people with blue eyes were smarter, quicker, and more likely to succeed. She followed this by giving blue-eyed students special classroom privileges. Brown-eyed children, she told the students, were lazy, stupid, untrustworthy, and inferior to blue-eyed boys and girls. To symbolize this, she made the brown-eyed children wear special ribbons and prohibited them from drinking out of the blue-eyed water fountain. She also lavished the blue-eyed students with praise and displayed more negativity toward the brown-eyed children.

In short order, Elliott was amazed to observe the blue-eyed children becoming bossy, arrogant, and unpleasant toward the brown-eyed students. Similar to the reaction of the prisoners in the Zimbardo study, the brown-eyed children became timid and intimidated. Even more remarkably, they began to show a decline in their academic performance while those with blue eyes excelled. Days later, she informed the children that she had made a mistake and that it was actually the brown-eyed children who were superior. As expected, roles reversed immediately. Elliott's experiment was captured in the documentary, *The Eye of the Storm*, in 1970 and later followed up by the 1985 *Frontline* episode, "A Class Divided," in which a number of these students reflect back on how the experience had affected their lives 15 years later.

One of the reasons why our behavior can switch rapidly in these circumstances is that social pressure to conform can be very powerful. In 1951, psychologist Solomon Asch recruited 50 male students from Swarthmore College to participate in a mock

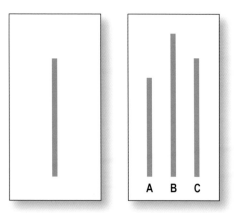

Figure 6.2
Perception lines

vision test (Asch 1955). In this test, each participant was placed in a room with seven confederates whose responses were determined in advance. The participant was led to believe that the other men in the room were also there for a vision test. This group of seven men and the real participant were presented with 18 trials in which they were asked to identify which one of three lines (a, b, or c) was longest in length (Figure 6.2). The confederates were pre-instructed to provide the incorrect answer on 12 of these trials. On average, nearly one third (32%) of participants concurred with the erroneous majority on the incorrect trials. Over the 12 trials, approximately 75% of the participants endorsed an incorrect response at least once. Later, when they were interviewed, participants stated that they were afraid of being perceived as odd or ridiculed if their answers were contrary to group opinion or that they assumed the group's answers must have been correct. In either case, the pressure to be accepted superseded the drive to respond correctly according to their perceptual experience.

In summary, we classify others according to our personal stories and mindsets. These stories are highly situational and contextual, often serving the function of maintaining connection to our social group. We are more likely to capitulate to social pressure or yield to authority and behave in ways that maintain our status in our group when faced with social rejection. In other words, we are susceptible to "groupthink" – the tendency to make irrational or dysfunctional decisions in the interest of maintaining conformity and harmony (Janis 1982). Imagine the consequences when we live in a chronically stressed, fearful society. As history tells us, the consequences can be devastating.

The Consequences of Bias

Systems and societies are comprised of humans. As we've seen, humans are subject to implicit biases, distortions, authority, and social influence. These influences can lead to altruism and kindness, as when millions of people around the world donate time and money to help others following a natural disaster or reach out to support political refugees. They can also spark fear, paranoia, discrimination, and horrific acts of cruelty.

When it comes to social engagement, we tend to possess positive attitudes about ourselves, and to those with whom we feel similarity. Conversely, we may create negative stories about dissimilar others (Banaji & Heiphetz 2010). Implicit bias refers to the relatively automatic and unconscious attributes of prejudiced judgment and social behavior. They reflect underlying stories or attitudes we hold about an object and its evaluation. Research into implicit bias emerged because scientists realized that people tended to be inaccurate in communicating their attitudes, in part, because they are driven to report what they think that they should feel, rather than what they believe to be true (Rudman 2004).

Implicit biases often develop based on our childhood environments, social learning history, culture, views of self, and affective experience. Promising research in the field of cognitive neuroscience suggests that implicit bias may be related to activity in the amygdala, which we know is associated with emotional experiences including fear conditioning (e.g. Phelps et al. 2000). For example, researchers asked a group of Caucasian participants to observe faces of unfamiliar black and white males while undergoing functional magnetic resonance imaging (fMRI) that targeted the amygdala – the brain's emotion processing center. They were also asked to complete a version of the Implicit Association Test (Greenwald , McGhee, & Schwartz 1998). Results showed that individuals who scored highly on indicators of implicit racial bias also tended to demonstrate greater amygdala activation when shown unfamiliar black faces, but not familiar black faces. This suggests that the amygdala's response to faces is related to a person's perception of a social group, but is also modified by knowledge and experience (Phelps et al. 2000).

Our personal stories tend to be laden with implicit bias. We may possess these biases even if we do not consider ourselves to be explicitly biased toward others. Although you may not think that biases affect your decision-making, your unconscious and conscious stories can, and often do, shape your social behavior in significant ways (Lieberman, Rock, & Cox 2014). In the social sphere, biases can affect behavior along many dimensions including a police officer's choice to shoot an alleged assailant, a physician's treatment plans, hiring determinations, legal verdicts and sentencing, and voter decisions, to name a few. They can also determine how you treat others on a daily basis (Rudman 2004). (You can take one or more Implicit Attitude Tests at Project Implicit – www.projectimplicit.com).

Although it may seem as though our implicit biases are relatively immutable, they can be influenced by external factors like technology. This impact may be positive or negative (Groom, Bailenson, & Naas, 2009; Peck et al. 2013). When it comes to spreading bias, digital information is a powerful tool that can rapidly shift the tide of public opinion. Information spreads across the globe in a matter of seconds, often before many of the details are accurately established. One terrorist act can immediately incite a global backlash against those perceived to be similar to the offenders. Not only that, but these assumed enemies are often vilified long before any verifiable information is known. In 1995, the Alfred P. Murrah Federal Building in downtown Oklahoma City, USA was bombed, killing 168 people and injuring more than 680 others, most notably children in a daycare center housed in the building. Within hours of the incident, news organizations were hypothesizing that Islamic radicals were responsible. No sooner was this news released than angry attacks were launched at Arab and Muslim civilians. Though this was prior to the 2001 World Trade Center bombing, memories of the 1993 bombing of the Center had produced a bias that Muslims and Arabs were most likely to launch another attack. It was later revealed that the bombing was the work of Timothy McVeigh, a white American and U.S. militia movement sympathizer.

Corporations are beginning to take notice of the impact of biases on decision-making. In the U.S. alone, companies are investing hundreds of millions of dollars per year on "diversity" and "sensitivity" training. These programs tend to yield marginal results, however. One of the potential reasons for this is that people often have little insight into their implicit thoughts, beliefs, judgments, and biases. In the paper, "Breaking Bias," Lieberman, Rock, and Cox (2014) suggest that our lack of awareness and refusal to accept bias are the biggest obstacles standing in the way of identifying and mitigating it. "This resistance to evidence of our own susceptibility, paired with the often-unconscious nature of cognitive bias, creates a perfect storm in which bias is perpetuated and rarely adequately recognized or managed," they write (p. 4). They believe that the most problematic issue in breaking bias is its unconscious nature and the "insidious" desire to be right. They propose three key steps to recognizing and addressing this problem. First, accept that people and systems hold biases that we are not aware of. Second, label biases based on the "underlying biology driving a particular bias." And third, mitigate bias by addressing core mechanisms that are underpinning that bias. As we've explored previously, lack of awareness and defensiveness are key features of highly-stressed individuals. When in states of physiological or psychological flooding, we are much less capable of insight and more likely to hold firm to our biases and rigid beliefs.

Moving Beyond Bias by Addressing Stress

Thus far, we have learned that chronic stress can inhibit our ability to attend to others mindfully in relationships, reduce our capacity to think, act, and communicate effectively, and damage our health and relationships. When in states of stress we are more likely to rely on our stories to interpret our social milieu, which can lead to biased, distorted, and rigid thinking. Systems are comprised of individuals who can lose their capacity for effective communication problem-solving and decision-making. They may defer responsibility to authority figures and adopt behaviors that protect their group status. As Lieberman and colleagues note (2014), it is critical that we recognize these influences if we are ever to successfully work with them.

As we discussed in Chapters 2 and 3, the first step in reducing the cycle of stress and its effects is to examine your life circumstances honestly. Consider the following questions.

Am I living in a state of chronic stress?

How well am I coping with the stressful circumstances in my life?

Are my personal or professional relationships impacted by how I cope with stress?

Is there something that I could be doing differently that would reduce my stress level and improve my relationships?

Part 2 of this Book

This book offers seven highly useful skills that will enable you to become more mindful in your relationships. Chapter 7 introduces you to the BREATHE model and explains why it is important and the research behind it. Chapters 8–14 take you on a step-by-step journey through each of the BREATHE tools, offering examples to inspire you on your journey. As you may have already gathered, this book does not advocate a single path or practice. Instead, it provides information regarding how our bodies and minds work and how each can sabotage the other, particularly when we are stressed and overwhelmed. I'm a big believer that knowledge is power. Understanding how our systems work is half the solution to becoming more resilient in the face of stressful life circumstances.

The BREATHE approach is an invitation. It is based on a large body of research in neuroscience, psychology, and psychophysiology, as well as a vast tradition of contemplative offerings that many have used as tools for personal transformation. This approach has been informed by science as well as observations from my work with adults, children, families, and groups who were suffering and looking for answers, and my own personal journey.

Whether you are new to these ideas or an experienced mindfulness practitioner, these tools are designed to encourage you to examine mindfulness not only as an intrapersonal journey, but also a relational one. In learning to care for ourselves, we can extend that offering to others and to the planet we inhabit.

PART 2

BREATHE

If you're reading these words, perhaps it's because something has kicked open the door for you and you're ready to embrace change. It isn't enough to appreciate change from afar, or only in the abstract, or as something that can happen to other people but not to you. We need to create change for ourselves, in a workable way, as part of our everyday lives.

Sharon Salzberg

7 | The BREATHE Model

Yesterday I was clever, so I wanted to change the world. Today I am wise, so I am changing myself.

Rumi

Breathing is essential for life. Yet most people are only vaguely aware of their breath the vast majority of the time. We appreciate that it speeds up when we exercise or work hard, and that we can halt it momentarily when we jump into water. But, for the most part, we are unaware of the relationship between how we breathe and our physical and mental experience. We are literally disconnected from one of our greatest resources!

You may wonder how the simple act of breathing can change your inner world and your relationships with others. After all, breathing is a solitary act. You don't need anyone else to breathe for you or tell you what to do. But if you pay close attention, your breath is a barometer of what is going on inside of you. When you're happy or content, your breath is slow, steady, and at ease. When you're anxious, irritable, angry, or threatened, your breath becomes shallow, rapid, or uneven. You may even notice your heart racing or your temperature rising.

In my many years working with clients, students, and workshop participants, I have observed one fascinating phenomenon. Most of us are not aware of our full breath capacity, and are largely unfamiliar with the breath's ability to modulate our experience. This doesn't apply only to those with asthma or chronic obstructive pulmonary disease (COPD). It applies to virtually everyone. The overwhelming majority of people inhale and exhale from the upper chest, leading to unnecessary work for the muscles of the neck and shoulders. A small proportion of others, like the athletes with whom I've worked, are able to draw breath into the lower reaches of their lungs, but often forcefully and at the expense of expanding the upper chest. Either way, an attenuated or forced breath cycle communicates to the brain and body that our system is under duress. As we learned in Part 1, the nervous system responds to perceived challenge by dumping stress hormones into our blood stream, increasing muscle tension, constricting blood vessels, cutting off blood supply to nonessential functions like digestion and reproduction, and priming us for aggression, avoidance, or withdrawal.

As we also learned in Part 1, chronic stress is associated with physiological hyper-arousal, or states of "flooding." When flooded, emotions and survival instincts take over, inhibiting the brain's capacity for planning, reasoning, and higher order communication. In this state, we are more likely to rely on self-defeating personal stories as lenses of perception, limiting our capacity to live in the present moment and interpret events mindfully. The repetition of negative personal stories undermines our health, happiness, and relationships, which magnifies the experience of stress.

The brain and body engage in a continuous feedback loop, each informing the other of the metabolic output necessary to cope with present circumstances. The breath is a primary participant in this loop. The more rapid or shallow the breath, the more we sense discomfort, tension, unease, and emotional instability. Conversely, when respiration is slow and steady, the parasympathetic nervous system (PNS) is activated, inducing the relaxation response and enhancing our ability to remain calm, present, and focused, even in the face of stressful life events (Elliott & Edmonson 2006).

Believe it or not, as you will see in the next chapter, you can literally shape your physical and psychological experience by altering your breath (Iyengar 1995; Jerath et al. 2006; Sovik 2000). Adopting breathing strategies that reduce physiological reactivity and induce relaxation affords you the space to turn down the volume of the unhelpful stories that play in your mind. These breath modification techniques, designed to balance the autonomic nervous system, are the most accessible and easy-to-learn strategies for reducing the physiological stress and its sequelae. When calm and centered, regions of the brain that govern thinking, planning, and reasoning are far more accessible, allowing for mindful awareness of thoughts, feelings, and actions.

Building Resilience One Breath at a Time

One of my teachers often repeated the phrase, "Pain is inevitable, suffering is optional." The first time I heard him utter those words, I was huddled under several blankets in my parka wearing multiple layers of clothing inside a poorly insulated retreat center in Northern California in December. In the pre-dawn darkness, I was sure that I was suffering. My fingernails were blue, I couldn't stop shivering, and it felt as though all of the muscle fibers in my body were contracted into balls of tightly wound knots. Although I understood that he was suggesting that suffering is a mindset, I couldn't think beyond my body's discomfort.

My teacher's words reminded me of those of William James, the highly influential nineteenth century American philosopher, psychologist, and physician often referred to as the "Father of American Psychology." James was an eternal pragmatist who believed that "the greatest weapon against stress is our ability to choose one thought over another" (James 1884). Similarly, Hans Selye, a twentieth century pioneer of stress research, also contended that resilience against stress could be enhanced by a positive attitude. He is well known for saying, "Adopting the right attitude can convert a negative stress into a positive one" (Selye 1956). But as I sat on the floor feeling cold, exhausted, and in pain, a positive attitude didn't seem possible. Even so, I began to wonder about this statement: "Pain is inevitable, suffering is optional." Was I causing my own suffering by feeling miserable about my circumstances? If so, how? How can we choose one thought over another when we are dealing with intense physical discomfort or psychological distress? Is it even possible to see the bright side of life when dealing with an onslaught of difficult events, or when engaged in conflict with others? Years of examining these questions and witnessing others courageously navigate their own personal and professional gauntlets have led me to believe that the answer is yes.

If we return to Selye's definition of stress as being anything that threatens our physical and psychological homeostasis, or balance, it is obvious that stress is unavoidable

(1956). But there is a flip side to stress, namely, resilience. Some people are more able to withstand or cope with life's repeated demands and maintain physical and psychological health, even when having to deal with stressful circumstances. The reasons for this are complex, involving a combination of individual differences in childhood experience, genes, cognitive functioning, mindset, emotion regulation, coping skills, and physiological reactivity (Dunkel Schetter & Dolbier 2011). Whatever the reason, there are those who possess a tremendous amount of grit from whom we can learn a great deal about resilience.

My aunt Grace, to whom this book is dedicated, is one such person. Margaret Grace Cini began her life humbly in 1921 as the daughter of poor, uneducated immigrants who fled the island of Malta after World War I. In her early life, Grace witnessed a great deal of pain and suffering. Her formative years were marked by the death of her father and older sister, Josephine, leaving her with a grieving mother and a younger sister, Georgina. Shortly after her husband's death, Grace's mother, my grandmother, married my grandfather, John, and had three more daughters. Several years after the youngest daughter, my mother, was born, my grandfather died of cancer.

Like most women of her generation, Grace got married and had several children, and her husband left to fight in World War II. By the time I was born, she was a single parent of three adolescent sons and a daughter, but no one ever spoke about her husband. After her death in 1995, I learned that she had left him to protect her children from his abusive behavior. In spite of the pain and hardship that my aunt endured, she possessed one quality that made her remarkable – grace. I never once heard her utter an ill word about anyone. Perhaps you could attribute that to her faith. She was a devout Catholic who attended mass at her local church every day. But I think that it was more than that. She embodied a fundamental belief in the goodness of others, and it showed in everything that she did. Stress and life experience didn't harden her or bleed into her relationships. She seemed to accept each experience as part of life, and cared for herself and others in the best way that she knew how. Whatever combination of resiliency factors she was dealt, she used them to make the world a better place. And she did it well.

As we learned in Chapters 2 and 3, it is difficult to harness the tremendous power of our minds and bodies or experience our resilient nature when stuck in a chronic stress feedback loop. But there is hope. Breath modification exercises like intentional breathing, which we will explore in the following chapters, can break this cycle and increase our capacity for awareness, insight, and effective coping.

The BREATHE Model

The BREATHE model is predicated on the assumption that the breath is the gateway to mindfulness. In using intentional breathing, you can balance the autonomic nervous system and reduce the stress response, usually within minutes. This increases your awareness of the experience of physiological and emotional flooding, and empowers you to defuse emotional reactivity and increase self-regulation.

In addition to its emphasis on recognizing and reducing physiological stress, the BREATHE model emphasizes the importance of examining the stories that shape your perceptions and behaviors. Familiarity with the ways that you use these stories to construe and construct your mental world allows you to recognize, appraise, accept, challenge, or refute them, rather than be governed by them. From here, you can enact decisions based on present events, rather than react from past wounds or future expectations. You become the empowered author of these personal narratives, and can rewrite them if you choose.

The BREATHE model also underscores the need for making a commitment to take time to care for yourself. Without dedicating even small amounts of time to breathe, rest, and engage in self-reflection, it can be difficult to enact sustainable life changes, particularly when life is stressful. Another key element of BREATHE is humor. One of the greatest deterrents to change is perfectionism. In many respects, it is a setup for failure. If you expect to be perfectly mindful all of the time, you are likely to be disappointed when you stumble and fall. You can avert suffering by holding yourself to the standard of doing the best that you can, and accepting your flaws and foibles. They are what make you human.

As stated in the title of this book, the BREATHE model is intended not only to be a tool for personal transformation, but also a vehicle for social change. Given the intimate relationships and interdependence that we share with family, friends, neighbors, co-workers, and the other inhabitants on this planet, it is important for each of us to initiate and participate in internal reflections and external dialogues that examine, "How am I (are we) contributing to the wellbeing of others and the planet?" In examining the larger social impact of your presence, you may improve the quality not only of your life, but also of those you touch.

The BREATHE model isn't magic. Like learning to ride a bike or speak a new language, it requires time, commitment, and practice. Having moved from a place of high stress, reactivity, fear, and strained relationships myself, and observing a metamorphosis in students and clients, I believe that it is worth the effort. I hope you will, too.

8 | Breath Awareness

Breath is the vehicle of consciousness and so, by its slow, measured observation and distribution, we learn to tug our attention away from external desires toward a judicious, intelligent awareness.

B.K.S. Iyengar

Recently, I was reminded of how the stress response has the potential to derail my ability to be calm, rational, and skillful. It was an unseasonably hot and oppressive day in the Pacific Northwest. At 2:00pm, the mercury was already tipping 100 degrees Fahrenheit, and the air was so dry that my mouth felt like it was filled with cotton balls. I needed something to drink. Lugging my overstuffed laptop bag, I joined a procession of business people, policemen, and retirees escaping the heat at a local coffee shop.

With frothy cold chai in hand, I made my way to my favorite table nestled in the back corner alongside a tall window. I'd spent many an afternoon there, tucked behind a wooden table away from the din of conversation, happily tapping away on my laptop keys. As much as I enjoy the company of others, there is sanctity in being able to write in a coffee shop uninterrupted. But that day, it was not meant to be. No sooner had I powered up my laptop than I heard the raving of an imposing, angry, 50-something man barreling toward me with coffee cup in hand. He was intimidating: well over six feet tall, with flaming red hair and a flushed face to match, dressed in dirty faded jeans and a rumpled t-shirt. He was having a hotly animated argument with his apparently absent mother, screaming obscenities and threats at the top of his lungs. I froze, hiding behind my computer screen, hoping that he would head for the back door several feet away. No such luck.

Before I knew it, he plunked down sideways in a chair at an adjacent table inches from my left shoulder and proceeded to read my computer screen. I could feel his hot breath on the back of my neck as he continued to rant. I was boxed into my once peaceful corner, unable to escape without bumping into him. "Can someone help?" I thought. The back of the shop was empty. No one seemed to be paying attention. He and I were the only two people within earshot. Not good.

My body immediately broke into sympathetic nervous system (SNS) overload. My heart raced like asynchronous rabbit paws drumming on a wooden deck. I broke out in a sweat as a primal fear flooded over me. I was trapped. As a relatively small person, my fear circuits overload when someone large and overpowering stands between an escape route and me. My gut buckled. I wanted to stuff my laptop into my bag, grab my drink, shove by him, and get out of there. But the little presence of mind that I had was telling me that bolting over him would likely inflame an already incendiary situation. Instead, I paused and took a breath – it was more like a gasp actually – but it was something. I asked myself whether I could find a mindful response to this situation. I practice and teach those skills, after all. But I had a big, irate man close enough to rub elbows and my nervous system was in overdrive. Could I find a way to calm down long enough to get a grip on my fear and respond thoughtfully rather than to freeze like a deer in headlights?

"Yes, I could," I told myself. I began to take deep, intentional breaths, inhaling and exhaling as slowly and fully as I was able. It took a few tries to move from near hyperventilation to long, intentional breathing, but once I fell into the calm rhythm of my breath, my sense of strength and composure returned. I closed my laptop cover, reached for my drink, and sat there, savoring the comforting taste of chai and the cool sensation of it flowing into me. I just sat – breathing, drinking, and, of course, observing my animated neighbor from the corner of my eye.

Then a strange thing happened. He stopped yelling. He heaved a big, audible sigh, picked up his coffee, and began to drink. Over the course of the next two minutes, I could feel his anger deflate. His posture shifted from imposing, angry, and agitated to slumped and defeated. In that moment, I felt my heart soften. "Excuse me miss," he said to me quietly. "Would you happen to have an aspirin? My sister just hit me and my head really hurts." I turned to face him. Unfortunately, I didn't have any pain relievers with me, but in my renewed state of calm, I did have the capacity to listen, and to treat him with kindness. He related that he'd had a really bad day and that his sister had hit him with her shoe. Just above his right eye, the skin was scratched and a welt was beginning to form. Between the heat and being slugged upside the head with a shoe, this poor man had indeed had a very rough go of it.

We spoke for a few minutes. He shared his sadness at having such a contentious family, and I listened and nodded, occasionally validating how difficult it must be for him. I suggested that we ask one of the employees for ice to keep the swelling down. He agreed. When I finished my drink and got up from the table, he thanked me for listening and wished me a good day. My heart softened a little more as I wished him one in return.

Our lives are full of opportunities to take a breath, slow down, and gain presence, even in very tricky situations. Some days, we respond with kindness and grace and, on others, our physiology and emotions get the best of us. Life is a practice, replete with moments when we can work on being kind to ourselves and others, and intentional breathing is a wonderful tool for disarming the stress response and creating space to respond to others differently. But we don't always know when we're in a state of physiological overload. In fact, for most of us, our constant state of stress makes it difficult to differentiate between having the capacity to cope with a challenging situation and needing to back off and regain our composure.

The Mechanisms of the Breath

Breathing occurs largely out of our conscious awareness. It is controlled by the autonomic nervous system (ANS) and is influenced by cells that monitor levels of blood gases like oxygen and carbon dioxide. The function of the ANS is to maintain equilibrium throughout the body's many systems to insure optimal functioning. Most of the visceral organs that are controlled by the ANS, like the heart and stomach, are made up of muscles that cannot be consciously controlled. But the lungs are different. They are comprised of spongy tissue and they rely on surrounding skeletal muscles, including the diaphragm, to function (Figure 8.1).

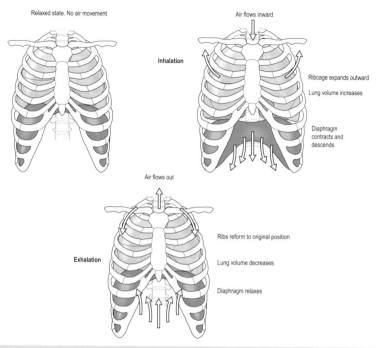

Figure 8.1

The mechanism of breathing

The diaphragm is the primary muscle responsible for facilitating breathing. It is a dome-shaped structure that sits just beneath the lungs, dividing the torso into two distinct compartments – the thorax and the abdomen. The diaphragm is controlled by the phrenic nerve, which originates between the third and fifth cervical vertebrae in the neck and descends between the lungs to each side of the diaphragm. This nerve is responsible for sending impulses to the diaphragm that tell it when to contract or relax based on the metabolic needs of the organism.

When the diaphragm contracts during inhalation, it draws the base of the lungs downward, causing them to expand, and the air pressure within them (intrapulmonary pressure) to fall below atmospheric pressure. This is what allows air to flow into the lungs. Airflow into the lungs ceases when the air pressure within the lungs is equal to atmospheric pressure. During exhalation, the diaphragm relaxes and moves upward, initiating the flow of air back out as the lungs shrink in size and the volume of the thoracic cavity decreases. This causes the air pressure within the lungs to rise above atmospheric pressure, and the air to leave the lungs until intrapulmonary pressure once again equals atmospheric pressure.

The impulses that control respiration originate in several regions of the brain (Guz 1997). Autonomic function, which controls the breath's automatic rhythm and maintains homeostatic balance, originates in the brain stem. Nerve impulses that allow you to volitionally control your breath – such as when you hold it while diving under water, blow out a candle, let out a forceful sigh, increase or decrease the volume of notes while singing or playing a wind instrument like a trumpet, or create audible words – originate in your cerebral cortex. Nerve impulses also come from the limbic system, the brain's emotional processing center. This is why your emotional state is intimately linked with the rhythm and quality of your breath.

Emotions significantly influence the mechanics of breathing (Homma & Masaoka 2008; Sovik 2000). Trip and nearly fall down or get startled during a film and you gasp in apprehension. Take in a beautiful vista and you may take in your breath in wonder. Laugh at a funny scene and your breath comes out in short bursts. When anxious or fearful, you may notice that you routinely hold your breath.

Stress also impacts the quality of the breath (Brown & Gerbarg 2005a, 2005b; Homma & Masaoka 2008; Sovik 2000). Similar to emotions, this influence may be situational, as when you're rushing to a meeting behind schedule, or become habitual when you are chronically in a stressed state. When under persistent stress, we often adopt unhealthy breathing patterns such as exaggerated movements of the chest or neck, tensing abdominal muscles, or breathing through the mouth instead of the nose. In time, these poor habits can be wired into the brain.

Just as stress and emotions contribute to dysfunctional breathing patterns, breathing patterns also influence our emotional experience (Fried 1999). Short, rapid, or exaggerated respiration causes anxiety, agitation, irritability, muscle tension, and a host of other problems that can ultimately contribute to chronic conditions and illness. This is why breath awareness is so vital to emotional wellbeing, including the health of our relationships. By observing the breath, we can quickly tap into our experience of stress or our emotional state, and use that information to make informed decisions about how we choose to respond (Elliott & Edmondson 2006; Brown & Gerbarg 2012; Sovik 2000).

Tuning in to Your Stress Level Through Breath Awareness

How do you know when it is no longer a good idea to keep pressing on with a difficult conversation? John Gottman's (2015) work suggests that as soon as your heart rate exceeds 100 beats per minute, you're already there. But most of us don't walk around with a heart rate monitor, so we need to rely on our own body wisdom. Unfortunately, very few of us know our body sufficiently well to accurately sense its state.

When I first began practicing yoga, and again when I began to incorporate body-based, somatic experiencing techniques into my work with clients, I was shocked by how disconnected most of us are from our bodies. Sure, we know when we're hungry, tired, in pain, whether our arms are raised, or if we're sitting or standing, but a small few of us are really tuned in to the amount of stress and emotional experience we carry in our physical bodies. This is due, in part, to the fact that our culture emphasizes intellect over physical or emotional intelligence. We're taught that we can think rather than feel our way through problems. In fact, feeling, or emotion, is often perceived as weakness, vulnerability, or the antithesis of intellect.

The truth is that our bodies are repositories of knowledge and experience. When we learn to harness that understanding through somatic awareness, we become better able to cope with stress and the demands of our relationships. Somatic awareness refers to our ability to feel and attend to external senses (sight, hearing, taste, touch, and smell), our proprioceptive experience (the sensing of our movements), and our interoceptive awareness (the sensing of physiological sensation within the body) (Levine 1997; van der Kolk 2015). It isn't easy or intuitive to tap into the body's experience if we're not used to paying attention to it. But it is a skill that can be learned.

Many common idioms and metaphors in the English language offer clues to how the body responds to stress. Consider the following phrases.

That made my blood boil.

I had butterflies in my stomach.

I was seeing red.

My heart sank.

I was on pins and needles.

I was shaking like a leaf.

I carry the weight of the world on my shoulders.

I'm full of beans.

I feel hot under the collar.

Keep a stiff upper lip.

I was gritting my teeth.

I poured my heart out.

I was all steamed up.

That struck a nerve.

I was on tenterhooks.

I was tongue-tied.

That tugged at my heartstrings.

I was weak at the knees.

Each of these phrases describes an experience that occurs when we are in an emotional state. Chances are you've experienced quite a few of them. What makes these expressions poignant is that they link emotions to physical sensations. As such, they provide important clues as to how our bodies react when we are feeling stressed or experiencing a particular emotion. Read back through the list and check off the items that you can most relate to in your experience of being stressed or emotionally upset.

Breath Awareness

As we explored in Part I, the breath is intimately connected to the stress response. As you become increasingly more aware of how you breathe, you will notice that the pace and depth of your breathing change depending on what you are thinking, feeling, or doing. It's all a matter of becoming aware of its patterns and fluctuations.

EXERCISE
Becoming Aware of Your Breath

The following practice introduces a simple yet effective technique to become attuned to your breath. The emphasis here is on observing how you breathe and beginning to become familiar with the breath's sensation. Remember that this is a practice. It may feel strange, awkward, or difficult, and you may or may not be able to sense a great deal at first. Don't worry. These feelings are common when you aren't used to sensing what is going on in your physical body. Be kind to yourself and remember that this is an exploration. Also remember that if, for any reason, you feel really uncomfortable or this doesn't feel right to you, take a break, and try again another time.

First, find a quiet place where you can sit for roughly 10 minutes without interruption. If you're worried about turning off your phone or shutting your spouse, children, dogs, cats, or other companions out of the room, don't be. They will be just fine without you for 10 minutes. Trust me, I've been there.

Now assume a comfortable position like sitting upright in a chair or lying on your back. If you're sleepy, I'd suggest sitting up or this may turn into a nap.

Begin to observe your breath just as it is. Notice where you are breathing into – upper chest, front, back, or sides. There is no right or wrong way to breathe – just observe for a few minutes. Once you get familiar with the flow of your breath, you may want to consider a few of these questions.

How does your breath feel as you breathe in and out? It is shallow or deep?

Is it easy to breathe or does it take effort?

Does your breath flow smoothly in and out or does it feel as though it gets stuck in some places?

Does it tend to move into the front or back or sides of your torso?

What is the pace of your breath? Does it seem typical or is it faster or slower than what you usually experience?

Has your breathing changed since you started observing it?

Do you notice any other sensations in addition to your breath?

Continue to observe the sensations for a few more minutes, noticing any feelings or thoughts that arise. Most importantly, try to become familiar with the rhythm and flow of your breath while remaining comfortable and relaxed. This may be the first time that you've paid much attention to the subtleties of your breathing. If it feels strange or you feel a bit anxious or uncomfortable, rest assured that your feelings are typical. Most new experiences make us uneasy.

Once you've spent three to five minutes becoming familiar with your breathing, pause, and take a break. Then reflect on some of the questions above and your experience. Did you learn anything new about your breathing or about yourself?

This exercise is very helpful for becoming familiar with the rhythm and sensation of the breath when you are calm and relaxed. It's almost like taking your physiological or emotional pulse. Once you gain familiarity with the sensation of your breath, you will start to notice changes more easily. When you feel yourself getting angry or agitated in traffic, in a meeting, or in the midst of a conversation, you may observe changes in your breathing pattern and the feelings associated with those changes. Rapid or shallow breathing is a sign that your SNS is reacting to a perceived threat. Once you've entered this aroused state, there's a good chance that your ability to be calm, rational, listen attentively, and respond skillfully is lowered, or lost altogether. This is an excellent time to take a break or to alert others that you need a pause.

Michael's Story

Michael is a successful, 54-year-old African American litigator who came to my office with concerns about his growing anxiety in the courtroom. He reported that he had "frozen up" during a recent trial. Seeing that Michael seemed unable to speak, the judge called for a recess. Michael was devastated. As a trial attorney, his living depended on his ability to perform in court and under pressure. His high-achievement orientation and integrity left him grappling with whether he could satisfactorily represent his clients. He was consumed by anxiety and feelings of inadequacy, guilt, and shame.

Having recently experienced a lot of turmoil at home, Michael doubted himself and his ability to "keep his anxiety under control." As his symptoms escalated, so did his fear and his fear story – that he was no longer competent to perform his job. Michael had a daily meditation practice and was an avid runner. By all accounts, he had good strategies in place to manage his stress and distress, yet nothing seemed to be working.

Michael and I began our work together using the same breathing exercise that we practiced above, and then built on it using the exercises in the upcoming chapters. Pretty soon, he was able to attain a sense of calm prior to entering the courtroom, which helped a great deal. But he still was afraid that the anxiety would "ambush him" when he least expected it. So we came up with a plan. We began to explore the physiological warning signs of trouble so that Michael could plan ahead in the event of an anxiety attack. We used the breath awareness exercise above and expanded upon it to include other warning signs that he was becoming flooded (see Chapter 9). In Michael's case, he often felt his skin "tingling" immediately prior to freezing. We worked on increasing his capacity to feel those signals by getting him in touch with his bodily sensations. Then we used intentional breathing to interrupt his cascade of symptoms.

Michael began to practice breathing and scanning his body for warning sensations before his meditation practice as well as many times throughout his day. By his next court appearance, he was prepared, albeit slightly apprehensive. Prior to entering the courtroom, he took several minutes to practice intentional breathing. By the time he appeared in front of the judge, he felt relaxed and confident.

During the next few months, I introduced Michael to several additional breathing practices, and we explored the personal narratives that contributed to his anxiety attacks. The last time I ran into him, he happily related that he had not had any more anxiety episodes in the courtroom. These successes have allowed him to unlearn his story that he was no longer competent to represent his clients, and he is again secure in his work and his career. What's more, he is taking on high stakes cases, assured that he has the skills to manage fear, anxiety, and self-doubt should they arise. He has continued his breathing practice, finding it to be a great addition to his daily meditation.

Michael's experience reminds us that not all problems are solved by thinking. This is particularly true when we are chronically stressed or our physiology and limbic systems are overriding our capacity for rational thought. In those situations, our bodies can, and often do, dominate our experience and we react rather than respond. Michael's story illustrates how practices like intentional breathing and scanning our bodies for physiological warning signs can be effective tools, even in the midst of high stakes professional interactions. Rather than entering the danger zone of stress, fear, anger, anxiety, or a host of other emotions that derail our capacity to interact skillfully, we can circumvent the process if we practice regularly and have these tools readily at our disposal.

If you look back on the story that began this chapter, you will notice that my encounter with an angry coffee shop patron was chock full of physiological cues that I had entered SNS overload and was struggling to keep my wits about me in the midst of a fight or flight response. To use some of the idioms and metaphors described previously, I was tongue-tied, gritting my teeth, shaking like a leaf, and most certainly weak at the knees. All of those cues, not to mention my racing heart and shortness of breath, were clear signs that I had to get my physiology calmed down before I could navigate the situation effectively. That is one tall order! In that instance, it was a matter of reading the signs and choosing the appropriate strategy to calm down. Since I use the breath often as a tool to get my nervous system back into balance, that was the first and easiest tool to grab out of my toolbox. It worked. A couple of minutes of breathing were all that it took to regain my composure and make an informed action rather than a hasty decision.

When we're agitated, anxious, or afraid, it can be very difficult to access these tools, which is why practice is so important. I believe that intentional breathing and scanning our bodies for signs of overload are powerful strategies because we can practice and use them anywhere, and they work – quickly. In the next chapter, we will continue to explore how to use intentional breathing to calm our physiology. In subsequent chapters, we will investigate other strategies for somatic awareness, understanding emotional cues, and examining our personal stories.

9 | Regulating the Autonomic Nervous System Through Intentional Breathing

Rather than allowing our response to an event affect our breathing, we can learn instead to let our breathing change our relationship to the event.

Cyndi Lee

Early last summer, my dog Beau – a sweet, amiable, sable and white Shetland Sheepdog – and I drove to a trail an hour out of town for a hike. It was a bright, clear July morning. The air was still and the mercury was rising swiftly toward a forecast high of 90 degrees Fahrenheit. Compact and low to the ground, Beau made easy work of the two miles of dusty trails that ascend above a creek, then wind down to the crystal water below. He dashed up and down the empty path, blissfully investigating a cornucopia of scents with a wide, contented grin.

As the temperature rose, so did the pace of his panting. My furry companion was feeling the effects of heat and clearly needed more than a few swigs from our water bottle to keep cool. So rather than wait for the path to level out alongside the creek, I took the next cut-off straight down a steep slope to the water. This meant a long, sharp descent through loose dirt and gravel that ended at the rocky shore below. Beau scampered briskly downward, eager to dip his angular little muzzle into the snow-fed creek. I did my best to navigate the hillside behind him. Before I knew it, I was flat on my back staring up the trunk of a massive Douglas fir tree. My feet had come out from under me, sending me airborne. My back slammed into the earth with such a jarring force that my teeth rattled. Somewhere during that aerial maneuver, I'd hit my head, leaving me dazed and disoriented.

Having broken my pelvis years before in an accident that left my lower body immobile for several months, my first thought was to see if I could move my legs. Check. Everything seemed to be in working order, albeit painfully so. I rolled over to pull myself up. A searing pain tore into my lower back like a hatchet blade jabbing into bone. "Ow!" I bellowed. "Ow!" the stone walls lining the creek echoed back. I was alone. We'd taken a lesser used trailhead because the path was blissfully untrodden most of the year – blissful until you're flat on your back, two miles from the road with no cell phone service and a concerned dog hovering over you. For the first time, I wished that someone else was behind us.

The pain was so intense that all I wanted to do was lie on my side and not move. But as I sized up the situation, I knew that I had no choice but to hike the two miles out to my car. I dragged myself onto my hands and knees, brushed the dirt from my catawampus sunglasses, and began to crawl back up the incline to the trail. The two miles of hiking back to the car were excruciating. I gasped for air with each step tread on the uneven stone and dirt path. I'm not sure how long it took us to get out, but it seemed to take forever. When we finally arrived home, I staggered up the stairs and made it to the couch where I passed out from exhaustion.

Mindful Relationships: Seven Skills for Success

In spite of how human brains have evolved to tackle complex problems, we haven't lost the primal instinct to stay alive. Thanks to my amygdala firing, and the hypothalamic orchestration of a symphony of stress hormones like adrenaline, cortisol, and norepinephrine, I had enough raw energy flowing through my veins to get me home. In this case, the fight or flight response was very adaptive. That changes when crisis becomes chronic. Then, these primal survival mechanisms become toxic. It's amazing to think that the very system designed to assure our survival can also be the ticket to our demise.

Sadly, chronic stress is a way of life. Many of us are so habituated to the exhaustion, pain, and dis-ease that come with persistent overload that we accept it as the norm. I fell into the ranks of the chronically stressed in my mid-twenties working as the director of business development for a successful architectural firm in Los Angeles. Year after year, I worked 70-hour weeks, fearful that I'd drop the ball on some important project or miss out on the opportunity for advancement. I sought refuge at the gym, where I'd punish myself with hard workouts, then end my days zoning out in front of the television. The more I pushed, the more my body pushed back. I suffered a series of illnesses, from adrenal failure to chronic fatigue. Asthma left me tense and gasping for air a great majority of the time. I felt depressed, anxious, trapped, and desperate. I tried psychotherapy and alternative medicine but still felt overwhelmed and burnt out a great deal of the time. My personal story – that I needed to work non-stop in order to survive – drove me like a relentless task master, never satisfied no matter how many hours I put in.

This pattern went on for nearly 20 years. I blamed my unhappiness on graduate school, then on my demanding career, and a failing marriage, fully believing that if I worked harder, succeeded professionally, and fixed my relationship everything would be fine. But it wasn't. My marriage eventually fell apart. Funding ran out and I lost my job. I had to face the harsh reality that working harder was not the answer. In fact, it only served to magnify my stress level and undermine my health and happiness. Then something happened that changed my life forever. I broke my hip.

At the time, I was so hyped up on stress and endorphins I didn't even know I'd fractured my upper femur. But when the orthopedist announced that I was at risk for never being able to walk properly again, I heard the wakeup call. Seven months on crutches with strict orders not to exercise were both the straw that broke the camel's back and the beginning of a cataclysmic shift. I lost my primary coping skills. All I could do was sit.

Somewhere in that stillness, I ran headlong into myself – confused, disillusioned, and suffering, spinning at such a high velocity that I couldn't see straight. I've watched many of my clients face this moment of truth; when the gaping hole between real and ideal is so great that you have to choose whether to fall into the abyss or find a different way of being. Those months of immobility did it for me. I was forced, kicking and screaming, to sit still and face myself. It wasn't pretty.

It wasn't the first time that I'd tried to sit still, but it was the first time that I had no choice. I'd tried meditation for several years, even spending a few weeks in a Zen monastery. No matter how hard I tried, sitting felt as unnatural as walking on my hands. I was so wound up that I could literally feel myself vibrating on the meditation cushion. Even though a part of me resonated with the experience of stillness, I could not quell the raging physiology that had me feeling like a cat on a hot tin roof.

Seven months on crutches felt like an eternity. By the time I'd been given clearance to exercise, a gentle yoga class felt like a life raft. I'd practiced yoga for a number of years, but at that time, it was just another form of cross training. I only attended challenging classes and never stayed through *savasana*, or "corpse pose," a period of time at the end of a yoga class spent lying on your back doing absolutely nothing. The thought of doing nothing didn't work for me. So I left while everyone else was "napping." I was a self-proclaimed *savasana* dasher!

Things felt very different after seven months of severely limited physical activity. I was grateful to do something…anything. I no longer felt the need to physically power my way through yoga class. Actually, I had so little leg strength or flexibility by that point that half the time all I could do was lie on my back and follow the breath cues. That's when the world shifted on its axis and I was introduced to a remarkable phenomenon. The breath.

Ninety minutes of intentional breathing and a bit of movement were transformative. My wound-up muscles relaxed – a sensation that was foreign to me at the time. I was no longer driven by a tyrannical mind demanding more. Within a matter of weeks, I enrolled in a yoga teacher training program. I was determined to figure out why mindfulness practices like yoga were so effective at reducing stress. If this could work for me, perhaps it would work for my clients, colleagues, and the other people that I knew who, like me, were chronically physically and psychologically stressed. If altering the breath in a yoga class led to reduced physiological hyperarousal and deep relaxation, what would happen if we breathed that way all of the time?

Breath and the Autonomic Nervous System

The breath is an amazing feat of biomechanical architecture. It is the only autonomic nervous system function that is unconscious but can be consciously controlled (Ley 1999; Sovik 2000). In essence, it operates not only as a thermostat, but also as a thermometer. As a thermostat, the breath changes in accordance with environmental demands, speeding up when you need to mobilize a response and slowing down when challenge has passed. As a thermometer, the breath's rate and depth feed information back to the nervous system, informing it about current physical and psychological states. For example, shallow, rapid breathing communicates to the nervous system that the environment is unsafe and that current metabolic resources are needed to combat a stressor. This is why you may feel uncomfortable, tense, irritable, or anxious when your breath is shallow. Conversely, you are more likely to feel calm and relaxed when the breath is deep and slow (Elliott 2006; Homma & Masaoka 2008; Iyengar 1985, 2004).

You may have observed that your breath is shallow and restricted to your upper chest when you're engaged in a stressful interaction. Shallow breathing is a response to stress that signals to the brain that it needs to mobilize to respond to a perceived threat. When breathing is consistently shallow, the mind–body system becomes stuck in a stress feedback loop. Shallow breathing, then, is both a sign and a symptom of chronic stress (Fried 1999; Sovik 2000). It is often accompanied by muscle tension, gastrointestinal upset, a clenched jaw, headaches, aggression, irritability, and even relationship conflict. Whether you're running from a gorilla, playing a violent video game, or imagining a worst-case scenario, it's all the same. The body and brain register stress and the breath cycle shortens. Because breathing is outside of our conscious awareness, we tend to give it very little thought. But our experience of breath reflects our experience of life, which is why breath awareness can be a very useful and important skill (Brown & Gerbarg 2005a, 2005b).

As we learned in Chapter 2, the sympathetic and parasympathetic nervous systems (SNS and PNS) are engaged in a continuous dance to maintain equilibrium. When in a state of homeostasis, both branches are in balance. The minute that a stressor is perceived, the vagal brake is released and the SNS becomes dominant to ensure survival. Once the threat has passed, the PNS takes over. Because the SNS responds instantaneously to threat, it is quick to activate and slow to disengage. Once activated, it typically takes a minimum of 20 minutes for muscle constriction to release and the flood of stress hormones to subside, assuming that danger is no longer present. Depending on the intensity of the stressor, it can take much longer. The PNS operates on a different timeline because relaxation is not essential to our immediate survival. Generally speaking, unless the vagal brake is applied, it takes longer for the PNS to activate and the relaxation response to be experienced. When stress is chronic, however, PNS activation is far less frequent (Porges 2011).

The breath is intimately connected with both SNS and PNS function. Inhalation is related to SNS activation (diaphragmatic contraction) and exhalation is related to PNS activation (diaphragmatic relaxation). This means that the autonomic nervous system (ANS) and the stress and relaxation response can be altered by manipulating the breath (Elliott 2006; Brown & Gerbarg 2009, 2012; Iyengar 1985; Sovik 2000). In the same way that shallow breathing amplifies the SNS, deep, intentional breathing, particularly slow exhalation, promotes PNS activation and vagal tone (Sakakibara & Hayano 1996). In a perfect world, we would feel relaxed and breathe deeply and fully more often than not. In reality, however, states of relaxation are often fleeting experiences rather than the norm. Most of my clients and students report being "stressed out most, if not all, of the time." If you stop to think about the implications, this means that most of us are at risk for heightened allostatic load and oxidative stress, not to mention physical and psychological dis-ease (Yoshikawa & Naito 2000). But you can do something about that by altering the rate and depth of your breath.

Intentional Breathing as the Gateway to Relaxation

The average adult takes approximately 10–20 breaths per minute depending on age, size, and health and fitness level. For the average person, this amounts to 21,600 breaths per day or about 600 million breaths in an 80-year lifetime! Stephen Elliot, yoga and martial arts instructor and author of *The New Science of Breath* (2006), contends that a respiration rate of 10 or more breaths per minute is correlated with "sympathetic dominance," or the tendency to be in persistent state of SNS activation. Sympathetic dominance is both a symptom and an indicator of chronic stress.

Both ancient and contemporary science of the breath show that PNS activation occurs during exhalation (Elliott 2006; Sovik 2000). When in danger or experiencing environmental challenge, exhalation is brief or shallow, and PNS activation is effectively "canceled out." Conversely, PNS activation can be stimulated by slowing down and deepening the breath (Sakakibara & Hayano 1996; Telles et al. 2013). The yoga tradition has long valued the practice of breath modification (*pranayama*) as a therapeutic tool (Iyengar 1985). Ancient yogis were acutely aware of the breath/autonomic nervous system/brain relationship and the potential for using intentional breathing to de-escalate the stress response and promote relaxation. They were also familiar with the breath as an autonomic feedback mechanism. According to renowned yoga teacher B.K.S Iyengar, "Emotional excitement affects the rate of breathing; equally, deliberate regulation of breathing checks emotional excitement. As the very object of yoga is to control the breath and still the mind, the yogi first learns *pranayama* to master the breath. This will enable him to control the senses and so reach the stage of *pratyahara* (the conscious withdrawal of the energy from the senses). Only then will the mind be ready for concentration" (Iyengar 2004, p. 48).

By far the most rapid way to initiate the relaxation response is through intentional breathing, which directly influences the ANS, including cardiac vagal tone and heart rate variability (HRV). Studies show that slow, intentional breathing decreases parasympathetic withdrawal (e.g. release of the vagal brake) in response to threat (Sakakibara & Hayano 1996). As breath deepens, exhalation slows, and as the number of breaths per minute decreases, the relaxation response increases (Ducla-Soares et al. 2007; Jerath et al. 2006). Intentional breathing, and resulting PNS stimulation, permits bodily systems (e.g. cardiovascular, gastro-intestinal, endocrine) to repair and regenerate. The relaxation response also reduces skeletal muscle contraction that often leads to muscle tension and pain (Benson, Beary, & Carol 1974).

Breath manipulation has been shown to have psychological effects including reducing the symptoms of anxiety, depression, chronic pain, post-traumatic stress disorder (PTSD), and other stress-related health conditions (Binello et al. 2016; Brown & Gerberg 2009; Elliott 2006; Rikard, Dunn, & Brouch 2015). The use of breath as a means for altering affect emerged because of the recognition of the reciprocal relationship between breathing and emotion. Specifically, emotional states are directly impacted by respiration and vice versa. This relationship between breath and psychological experience is becoming increasingly more recognized in the West. According to a national study, of the 2.9% of Americans who report using some form of mind–body therapy such as yoga, tai chi or Qigong, 84.4% practiced deep-breathing exercise – more than yoga and meditation combined (Nerurkar et al. 2011). This is likely due to the fact that breath modification is a relatively simple, accessible, cost-effective alternative for providers and patients looking to reduce stress.

Taking a deep breath or two in and of itself isn't new. Many people take a few deep breaths when they've feeling overcome by stress, and the adage, "just breathe" appears on everything from billboards to t-shirts. Deep breathing, often referred to as "belly or diaphragmatic breathing," is incorporated in many different therapeutic modalities and mind–body therapies. There is one fundamental problem with breath modification techniques, however. The majority of people are not fully aware of their lungs' capacity. Consequently, they fail to inhale or exhale fully. Why is this the case?

A great many individuals are disconnected from the sensations and feedback from their bodies. This absence of somatic awareness may be a result of life experience, such as trauma, or of living in a culture that reveres intellect and has embraced a medical model in which body and mind are divided rather than being considered holistically. In the years that I have been teaching breathing techniques, I have witnessed many clients, students, and workshop participants marvel at the discovery of their full breath capacity. Not convinced? Here's a fun exercise. Inhale deeply and then measure the length of your slowest possible exhalation. Now do it again, but this time, measure the duration of your exhalation as you sing "om" in a single note as slowly as possible. Did you find a difference?

EXERCISE
Intentional Breathing

The following practice introduces a simple yet effective form of deep breathing called intentional breathing. Unlike other techniques of "belly" or "abdominal" breathing, the emphasis here is to allow the natural flow of the breath by inhaling from the top down and exhaling from the bottom up. Before you begin, there are a couple of things to remember:

First, this is a practice. It may feel strange, awkward, or difficult. That is to be expected when trying something that you've never attempted before. Be kind with yourself and see this as an exploration rather than something to be immediately mastered. Second, and more importantly, if for any reason you feel really uncomfortable or this doesn't feel right to you, it is perfectly OK to take a break or discontinue the exercise and try again another time.

Begin by finding a comfortable position like sitting upright in a chair or lying on your back. Begin to observe your breath just as it is. Notice where the breath flows – upper chest, lower belly, front, back, or sides. As you do, try to avoid placing a judgment on how you are breathing or attaching a story to it. Just as if you were a scientist studying a cell under a microscope, see if you can examine all of the details of your breath one at a time and make mental notes of them.

Observe how you are breathing just as you are. It's an interesting exercise. You may already notice that the act of observing your breath slows down your respiration rate.

Next, place your right hand on your breastbone (sternum) in the center of your chest.

Place your left hand so that your thumb is below your navel. Continue to breathe normally and observe whether you are breathing more into your right hand or left hand. See if you can resist the urge to change your breath or make it deeper. Breathe as normally as you can and observe how it is to be in your body, breathing normally. How does it feel? What do you notice? Continue for at least 10 breaths.

Now try breathing just into your right hand that is resting in the middle of your upper chest. Without forcing the breath, see how it feels to breathe into the space below your right hand. What do you notice? Can you slow your inhalation or is that difficult or uncomfortable? Just see what happens. Keep observing for 10–20 breaths. After 10–20 breaths, take a few deep inhalations and exhalations and resume breathing normally for a minute or so.

Next, try breathing just into your left hand that is resting on your lower abdomen. Without forcing the breath, see how it feels to breathe into the space below your left hand. What do you notice? Can you slow your inhalation or is that difficult or uncomfortable? Just see what happens. Keep observing for 10–20 breaths. After 10–20 breaths, take a few deep inhalations and exhalations and resume breathing normally for a minute or so.

Now, try breathing half of your inhalation into your right hand, pause for a second or two, then breathe the remainder into the space below your left hand, and pause. Then exhale from the bottom up, first releasing the air below your left hand, then allowing the exhalation to continue from below your left hand to below your right hand, traveling up and out either through your nose or mouth. Continue to your next inhalation, first into the area beneath your right hand and then into the area beneath your left hand, then exhale from the bottom up. Can you slow your inhalation or is that difficult or uncomfortable? How does it feel? What do you notice? Keep observing for 10–20 breaths. After 10–20 breaths, take a few deep inhalations and exhalations and resume breathing normally for a minute or so.

Finally, try breathing deeply and fully from top to bottom as you inhale and bottom to top as you exhale, without pausing. If possible, see if you can slow the exhalation so that it is longer than the inhalation. If you like, you can count 1, 2, 3, and so on to see which is longer: your inhalation or your exhalation. After 10–20 breaths, take a few big deep inhalations and exhalations and resume breathing normally for a minute or so.

Notice how you feel. Was the exercise simple or difficult? Did breathing slowly and fully seem usual to you? How do you feel physically? Emotionally? Energetically? If you like, write down your experience.

This exercise is intended to activate your PNS and elicit the relaxation response. While not everyone experiences relaxation right away, most report feeling a sense of calm and a reduction in the feeling of stress after this exercise. Now, for fun, take in a deep breath and try singing "om" using a single tone again and count how long you hold the tone. Do you see a difference? Most people do!

Although most find this intentional breathing exercise to be beneficial and informative, it doesn't always work for everyone. Some people find it difficult to remain focused on the breath when their brain is in a constant state of chatter. One of my recent course attendees, Shirley, reported that even though the exercise was soothing, she struggled to keep her overactive mind in check. Her experience isn't uncommon. There are many strategies to work with the mind in this situation, but the one that seems to work best for most people is to attach their breath to a word or a phrase to keep the mind focused. Shirley, for example, slowly recited the words "in" with the inhalation, and "out" with the exhalation. Some eastern traditions suggest the words "so" on the inhalation and "hum" on the exhalation. Pretty much any word or phrase can work to help focus the mind on the sensation of the breath. The trick is to keep the word or phrase simple so that the experience is still centered on the somatic, felt, or body sense of breathing rather than the thought sense, or a word or story that describes it.

Regardless of what works for you, intentional breathing takes practice. The good news is that it can be practiced virtually anywhere and even when you are interacting with others (except when driving a car or operating heavy machinery, please). The more that you practice, the easier becomes. Particularly at the beginning, I suggest practicing intentional breathing at least a few times a day, every day, preferably in a quiet space and with all external distractions removed. You can do it whenever you find yourself sitting still for a few moments. It is much easier to learn a new skill while focusing on it, rather than trying to adopt it while multitasking.

Most of my clients and students report feeling benefits from this practice right away. They feel more calm and relaxed after a few minutes of intentional breathing. Over time, you may notice a shift in your awareness of your breath, or a tendency to breathe more deeply and fully most of the time. This is the first step in defusing the stress feedback loop and teaching your brain and body to relax.

10 | Experiencing Emotion

Be patient toward all that is unsolved in your heart and try to love the questions themselves… Live the questions now. Perhaps you will gradually, without noticing it, live along some distant day into the answer.

Rainer Marie Rilke

It's 3:00 PM on a summer afternoon when the unthinkable happens – my cat knocks a full glass of lemonade onto my laptop. I'd been glued to my screen writing since early that morning. It was sweltering outside and ice-cold lemonade seemed like just the ticket. No sooner did I return to my desk when I was joined by my fifteen pound, black panther of a cat named Arjuna. Arjuna is an affectionate, powerful cat that has no concept of his size and strength. Unfortunately, this means that he can inadvertently clear off my desk if I don't thwart his jumping up in time.

Engrossed in my work, I didn't catch him before he leapt onto a stack of articles, lost his footing, and skidded feet first across my desk. Before I knew it, he'd knocked the glass of lemonade over, sending the sticky yellow liquid into the keyboard. In one fell swoop I grabbed my laptop, flipped it over, and began tapping it like I was burping a newborn. In spite of my love for my cat, at that moment I was livid. My heart pounded frantically in my chest. My blood boiled. I could feel a rage rising up from my gut to my ears like a red tide about to burst its banks. I wanted to scream. Arjuna just sat there, staring contently at me with a big green gaze of feline indifference. In that moment I could have killed him. Well, not really, but you get the picture.

After consulting the technicians at my local computer store, I placed the sticky machine upside down on a towel atop a large milk crate above a small fan to begin the lengthy process of drying it out. The technicians said that I should not attempt to turn on my computer for a minimum of 72–96 hours. That's minimum of THREE DAYS before I knew whether or not my hard drive had been damaged. Three days of imposed silence to a writer in the middle of a project is the worst form of hell. I had clients, articles and a book to write, and deadlines. Anxiety welled up in my chest like a water balloon compressing the air out of my lungs. How would I cope without my computer? For many, three days without a laptop may seem like a much-needed holiday. To me, a writer, three days of cat-imposed exile from my work, notes, research, musings, calendar, and pretty much everything else felt like being thrown into oblivion.

Before learning to practice intentional breathing, I would have screamed at the cat, kept my computer on and tried to will it back to life, cried or ranted for hours, and been inconsolable. I also would have indulged my story of being incompetent because I had failed to prevent the situation. This time, I was able to recognize my stress, anger, and panic and find constructive ways of addressing or quelling these reactions rather than have them control me and potentially cause harm.

The first step in dealing with intense stress and emotional reactions is to breathe, deeply and fully (intentional breathing) until you begin to sense a shift into a less reactive state of mind. This can take several minutes depending on how wound up you are. The next step is to recognize the emotions and the bodily sensations that arise in response to your circumstances. In my case, the heat rushing to my face and pounding heart were telltale signs that my anger was reaching a boiling point. Because I'd created a bit of space for myself by pausing for a few moments of intentional breathing, I was able to grab the wheel of what felt like an out of control emotional skid and right its course. Breathing gives you the space to recognize the bodily sensations that arise in response to particular emotions, and empowers you to make a choice whether to act on these emotions or choose a different course. It isn't simple or easy at the time, but it can save a relationship from enduring the harm of an emotional outburst.

In her book, *My Stroke of Insight: A Brain Scientist's Personal Journey*, author Jill Bolte Taylor tells of her journey of recovering from a devastating stroke (Bolte Taylor 2009). In it, she describes the biological underpinnings of emotion including the fact that, in the case of an acute stressor, the physiological rush of cortisol, adrenaline, and other stress hormones is over within 90 seconds of the triggering event. When it came to my lemonade-soaked computer and smug cat, the only thing perpetuating my anger and anxiety was the story that I continued to tell myself about work that I wasn't attending to, my fear of not completing assignments on time, and what a stinker my nonchalant cat had been. Had I become stuck in that story, my anger would have persisted. Instead, once I calmed the stress response, I was able to identify my physical and emotional sensations and move beyond them, rather than wasting a lot of energy fretting over an unfortunate incident that had already occurred.

It can be very difficult to calm down and sit in a zone of discomfort when we are angry or feel harmed by others. Many times a quick attack or defense strategy seems like the best course of action. We've learned in previous chapters that when our systems are flooded with stress hormones and primed for battle, we are not in the best position to choose a rational response. When in doubt, bodily sensations like a racing heart, flushes of heat, trembling, shortness of breath, nausea, and muscle tension serve as important cues that we are anxious, angry, and ungrounded. This signals the need to pause rather than react hastily or mindlessly.

Where do Emotions Come From?

Although intervening at the level of the stress response is helpful, it can be difficult to regulate our emotions, particularly when they are powerful like grief or rage, or if we feel as though we have no control over them. The origin of emotional experience has been the subject of debate for well over a century. Formal conversation about the nature of emotion began in 1884 with an article written by the famous psychologist and philosopher, William James, entitled, "What is an Emotion?" (1884). In the article, James proposed that emotional experience both arises from, and is accompanied by, changes that occur in the body in response to a stimulus. Physiological reactions such as a racing heart, sweaty palms, tense muscles, and butterflies in the stomach are fed back to the brain via afferent (to the brain) channels in the nervous system.

James believed that emotions weren't processed until these afferent signals were received by the brain and perceived as emotion. In James' words, "My thesis … is that bodily changes follow directly the *perception* of the exciting fact, and that our feeling of the same changes as they occur *is* the emotion" (James 1884, p. 189). In other words, the sensory perception of the body is what gives rise to emotional experience. Although James acknowledged the role of appraisal in the experience of emotion, he saw it as secondary following the discernment of physiological arousal. In spite of the fact that James' theory was later dismissed due to its simplicity, he illuminated the importance of bodily input in emotional experience.

Several decades later, Walter Cannon, a renowned experimental physiologist, put forward an opposing theory (Cannon 1927). Cannon believed that emotions occur within the brain and do not rely on contributions from the body. Although he concurred that sensory information helped to shape affective experience, he contested the presumption that emotion was solely a function of visceral input. His thalamic theory of emotion maintained that the thalamus and hypothalamus produced the bodily sensations that the brain processed as emotional experience. His work, which centered largely on the function of the autonomic nervous system in animals and its role in intense feelings like anger and hunger, made an important contribution to our understanding of the sympathetic nervous system and the fight or flight response. It should be noted, however, that Cannon's assumptions were largely based on animal research.

Cannon's theory was widely accepted until 1937 when James Papez, a Cornell University professor of neuroanatomy, discovered the Papez Circuit, subsequently renamed the limbic system (Papez 1937). This circuit linked centers in the brain including the amygdala, prefrontal cortex, hippocampus, and cingulate gyrus. Although at that time researchers did not have sophisticated imaging techniques and based their assumptions on animal models, the work of James, Cannon, Papez, and others opened the door for subsequent investigations that showed that emotion is a mind-body phenomenon, involving both neurological and hormonal input ascending from the body to the brain and feedback from the brain to the body. In the words of Elmer Green, a physician and a pioneer in the use of biofeedback, and his colleagues, "Every change in the physiological state is accompanied by an appropriate change in the mental emotional state, conscious or unconscious, and conversely, every change in the mental emotional state, conscious or unconscious, is accompanied by an appropriate change in the physiological state" (Green, Green, & Walters 1979, p. 132). Indeed, contemporary research examining the conjoint influence of mind, body, and brain on emotional experience supports this proposition, suggesting that centrally integrated feedback from the body plays an important role in our perception of emotion (Damasio, 1999; Weins 2005).

The HeartMath Institute was founded in 1991 with the mission of bringing "physical, mental, and emotional systems into alignment with the heart's intuitive guidance." Part of this mission involved scientific studies of the heart–brain relationship. These investigations have yielded some interesting results, the most surprising of which is that the brain isn't the master controller of our beings as we once assumed. The heart actually sends more signals to the brain than the brain sends to the heart. Not only that but, as we saw in Chapter 2, by way of the vagus nerve, the heart and other visceral organs directly impact brain function including emotional experience and our capacity to engage in skills like problem-solving, attention, perception, and memory (McCraty 2015a, 2015b).

Studies conducted by HeartMath Institute scientists suggest that the heart is a remarkable indicator of our emotional state. When we are stressed, angry, aggressive, or experiencing other negative emotions, our heart rhythms become irregular. In addition, the limbic system inhibits higher order brain functions necessary for planning, reasoning, skillful action, and effective decision-making. This then feeds forward to perpetuate further negative emotional states and perceived stress. Like sympathetic nervous system (SNS) overload, irregular heart rhythms contribute to a mind–body–brain stress feedback loop, reinforcing our stress level and its negative impact. Conversely, peaceful emotional states contribute to synchronous heart rhythms, relaxation, and cognitive coherence (see McCraty 2015a for a review).

Although there is still a lot to be learned, it is clear that the heart plays a significant role in emotional experience. First, it maintains considerably more afferent projections to the brain than any other visceral organ, meaning that it sends more signals to the brain than other organ bodies. Second, the heart is highly sensitive to changes in autonomic input, and its rhythm shifts rapidly in response to changes in our internal and external environments. These shifts are readily detectable by most people. Because of this, we are often attuned to our heartbeat and its link to our emotional state. When experiencing intense emotion, we become aware that our heart rate is rapid, or pounding which may, in turn, feed back to our experience of stress, anxiety, fear, aggression, or other negative drives (McCraty 2015a, 2015b).

Considerable research supports the link between cardiac arrhythmias, decreased heart rate variability (HRV), respiratory sinus arrhythmia, and anxiety disorders (Licht et al. 2009; Fleet & Beitman 1998; Friedman & Thayer 1998). Studies of individuals with panic disorder, a condition characterized by sudden and repeated attacks of fear accompanied by physiological symptoms like a racing heart, shortness of breath, sweating, and dizziness, find that panic is often the result of the unexplained onset of cardiac arrhythmia. In one study, more than two thirds of patients with panic disorder reported sudden onset arrhythmias concurrent with developing panic. In most cases, panic attacks remitted or disappeared once the arrhythmia was diagnosed and treated (Lessmeier et al. 1997).

We can learn a lot about our bodies and emotional experiences by listening to the rhythm of our heart. Many of us are more aware of our heart rate than our breath because of its rhythmic quality, and its ability to noticeably change with activity or intense emotions like fear, anxiety, and anger. This is why your heart's rhythm can be used as a tool for tapping into your emotional experience and the sensations of being emotionally flooded. In becoming familiar with your resting heart rate and rhythm you can begin to detect when it is changing and, perhaps, when you are reaching a state of physiological flooding. Take a moment to try this exercise below and become a bit more familiar with your heart rhythm.

> **EXERCISE**
> **Experiencing Your Heart**
>
> Place one or both of your hands over your heart (on your chest to the left of your breastbone). Close your eyes or cast your gaze downward away from distraction.
>
> Take a few moments to see if you can feel your heartbeat. This may be easy or difficult depending on your familiarity with your body. Once you find it, observe the beating of your heart just as it is. What do you notice?
>
> Does your heartbeat seem fast or slow?
>
> Is it pounding or beating calmly?
>
> Is your heartbeat regular or irregular?
>
> Does it speed up, slow down, or maintain a consistent pace?
>
> Is there anything else that you notice about it?
>
> Take a few moments to write down your experience.

Interoception: Attuning to the Body's Messages

In many respects, James and Cannon were on to something. Even though their perspectives differed, they both acknowledged the role of bodily feedback in the experience of emotion. We now know that neural signals from the body's visceral organs, including the heart, lungs, and gut, are continuously transmitted to the brain. Interoception refers to the process through which the central nervous system interprets information from the body and uses it to generate conscious perception of bodily events (Schultz & Vogele 2015). Studies show that interoception and our experience of emotion are highly interconnected, such that bodily sensations can and do shape our mood (Barret et al. 2004; Critchley et al. 2004; Damasio 1999; Pallatos, Gramann, & Schandry 2007; Schultz & Vogele 2015; Wiens 2005).

One example of this is hunger. Hunger represents the physiological need for nourishment. It is driven, in part, by signals that come from the gastrointestinal (GI) tract upward through the vagus nerve to the brain. When we are hungry, we feel a desire to eat. When that desire is not met, we feel discomfort that can impact our mood. Infants, who are wholly dependent upon caregivers for nourishment, cry when they are hungry. Many adults that I know (including myself) get progressively grumpier the longer hunger persists. The hunger signals that travel from your gut to your brain can, and do, affect your mood. Now imagine if there was something inhibiting or preventing that signal. In the extreme, if you never had a desire to eat, you would eventually starve to death. The signal that your body sends to your brain creates motivation for action.

Neuroscientific research is helping to tease apart how interoceptive processes influence our subjective experience of emotions and stressors (Haase et al. 2015; Terasawa, Fukushima, & Umeda 2013). For example, a recent study of 46 adults who were divided into low, normal, and high resilience groups based on responses to a self-report resiliency survey, found strong links between resiliency and interoceptive awareness. Functional magnetic resonance imaging (fMRI) brain scans of these same individuals, taken while they completed an attention task where their breathing was intermittently restricted via a mouthpiece and a nose clip, showed that participants in the low resilience group had less interoceptive awareness, reduced attention to bodily cues, and higher levels of neural processing of aversive physical stimuli than those with greater resilience (Hasse et al. 2015). This means that individuals with lower levels of body awareness may be more susceptible to stress compared to those with greater body awareness. Intentional breathing is one tool that may enhance interoceptive ability by cultivating awareness of the breath and the physical sensation of breathing.

The Body Has a Mind of its Own

Interoception may also play a direct and important role in perception. Dr. Dean Radin is an author, senior scientist at the Institute of Noetic Sciences, and a pioneer in the field of parapsychology. Parapsychologists explore psychic and paranormal activities such as precognition, clairvoyance, telepathy, and apparitions. Although often considered a "pseudoscience" because methods and means of inquiry can fall outside the realm of acceptable scientific convention and rigor, pseudoscientists attempt to explain what conventional research often considers unexplainable, raising provocative hypotheses regarding the human experience.

Radin was one of the first to propose that our bodies can unconsciously anticipate future emotional states. In a study conducted in 1997, he measured changes in skin conductance, heart rate, and blood pressure in a group of adults as they were shown a random series of images on a computer monitor. These images included landscapes, disturbing images (autopsy photos), and arousing (erotic) pictures. Participants registered a physiological response before (rather than immediately after) viewing each photo. These reactions were most pronounced prior to viewing disturbing or erotic images (Radin 1997). This indicates that individuals may have an underlying, subconscious capacity to anticipate emotional states even before they occur.

To further understand this phenomenon, Dr. Rollin McCraty, director of the HeartMath Institute, collected detailed brain and heart readings of participants undergoing Radin's image viewing protocol. He found that both the brain and the heart registered responses prior to viewing the images. What's more, the heart reliably responded before the brain, raising the possibility that the heart may provide input that the brain uses to process environmental stimuli (McCraty, Atkinson, & Bradley 2004). Later studies revealed that reactions were also registered in the gut, somewhere along the lines of a gut feeling or gut intuition (see Mossbridge et al. 2014 for a review and critique of the research). This phenomenon, referred to as predictive anticipatory activity, insinuates that perception may not only be a mind–body phenomenon, but also occur beyond conscious awareness, and that input from visceral organs, like the heart and gut, may affect experience more than previously assumed (Mossbridge et al., 2014). Although this topic of research is not without its controversy, it raises the interesting proposition that human perception may be as much an embodied journey as it is a mental one.

Body Mapping Emotions

Emotions are as much experiences of the body as they are of the mind. They help to coordinate our behavior and physiological states during both stressful and pleasurable circumstances. Research suggests that individuals who are more accurate in their interpretation of bodily states report greater intensity of emotional experience than those who are less somatically aware (Barrett et al. 2004). This suggests that interoceptive skill may be an important contributor to understanding our emotional experience and also may enable us to exercise greater self-awareness when interacting with others.

Studies are beginning to offer insight into where particular emotions are felt in the body. This information may allow us to better understand the relationship between emotional experience and distinct physical sensations. For example, a group of Finnish researchers investigated whether discrete emotional states are linked to sensations in particular bodily regions (Nummenmaa et al. 2014). They invited 302 adult participants (261 female, mean age 27 years) into the laboratory where they were asked to view emotional or neutral words one by one. After seeing each word, the participant was asked to note where they felt physical sensation, and to digitally paint that bodily region on a computer image of an anatomically neutral human silhouette using a computer mouse.

Emotional words fell into one of three categories: "basic" (anger, fear, disgust, happiness, sadness, and surprise), "nonbasic" (anxiety, love, depression, contempt, pride, shame, and envy), or neutral. The digitally painted images were averaged across the entire sample, and then used to create silhouette drawings of "heat maps" that illustrated where each emotion was most frequently felt in the body. Finnish and Swedish (European) as well as Taiwanese (Asian) participants were included to test whether emotional body mapping was culturally specific.

The researchers then recruited a new sample of 72 adults and asked them to match each heat map with one of the basic or nonbasic emotion words that they felt best described the image. These responses were compared with the words that they gave the original sample to see how accurately the second group matched the emotion words to the body maps. For basic emotion words such as anger, fear, disgust, happiness, sadness, and surprise, participants were accurate in identifying the relevant area on the "heat maps" an average of 72% of the time. They were similarly accurate in identifying nonbasic emotions (anxiety, love, depression, contempt, pride, shame, and envy), but less so when trying to discriminate between emotions. The researchers found no differences by language or ethnic group, suggesting that human mapping of emotions onto bodily sensations may be universal. They also discovered that patterns of bodily sensation and their relation to emotion words were consistent with prior research regarding how emotions affect us physiologically. For example, most basic emotions like anger, fear, happiness, and sadness were mapped as being felt in the upper chest area. These are likely to correspond to increases in heart and breathing rates that we often notice when experiencing intense primary emotions. Sensations in the upper body and arms were most pronounced for feelings of happiness and anger, whereas less activation in this area was associated with sadness. This makes sense in light of recent research that demonstrates a direct relationship between slumped posture and feeling sad or fearful versus upright posture, which was related to strength, joy, and enthusiasm. The body maps also consistently identified the head as an emotional center, inferring that emotions such as anger, happiness, love, fear, disgust, and surprise are registered as facial expressions and/or mental events (Nummenmaa et al. 2014).

Taken together, emergent body mapping research suggests that interoceptive awareness may play a key role in understanding emotional experience. From a mindfulness perspective, in cultivating attentional awareness of our physical sensations such as an accelerated heart rate, a clenched jaw, a flushed face, furrowed brow, tight upper body, or stomach upset, we may gain insight into our emotional world. This may be especially useful when engaged in interactions with others, particularly when we feel physiological arousal or flooding. Intentional breathing, which fosters an awareness of the connection between somatic events and physiological and psychological experiences, is a first step in developing this awareness of bodily states.

EXERCISE
Attuning to Your Body

The following exercise uses intentional breathing to attune to where you may hold emotions in your body. Remember that this is a practice. It may feel strange, awkward, or difficult, and you may or may not be able to experience your emotions as bodily sensations. This is not unusual. We are often disconnected from the experience of our physical bodies, so it can take time and practice to develop that awareness. Remember that this is an exploration. If for any reason you feel uncomfortable or need to discontinue this exercise, take a break, and come back to it at another time.

First, find a quiet place where you can sit for roughly 10 minutes without interruption. Find a comfortable position sitting upright in a chair or lying on your back. If you're sleepy, I recommend sitting. Once you are comfortable, begin to breathe intentionally as you've practiced previously. Breathe into the heart area first and then down into the abdomen as fully and deeply as you are able, then exhale slowly, as if you are deflating the air out of a balloon from the bottom up. Once you find a comfortable rhythm, observe your breath for another few minutes as you move into a deeper state of relaxation.

Once you are breathing comfortably, shift your attention to your body. How does your body feel overall? What do you notice? Are there places where you feel tension or restriction? Are there areas of your body that are more relaxed? Are there any sensations that you feel more strongly? Focus your attention on whatever sensation you feel most strongly in your body right now. It may be very subtle or quite noticeable. Where is the sensation located? Once you've identified a location, give it your full attention for a few minutes.

Then shift your focus to the quality of that sensation. Can you find words to describe it like sharp, dull, tight, loose, stiff, throbbing, hot, cold, uncomfortable, or painful? Does this sensation remain in one place? Does it shift or change? See if you can keep your mind on the sensation and resist the urge to create stories around it. Notice how it feels and allow that feeling to be present without trying to alter it or describe it beyond a few words. What happens when you stay focused on that sensation for a while? Is there anything else that you notice about it? Do other sensations arise as well?

Then notice whether you feel any particular emotions while focusing on that sensation. As we learned above, our bodies store a great deal of information, often providing messages and clues about how we are feeling. What emotion or emotions, if any, do you feel when focusing in on that sensation? Remember, there are no right or wrong answers. You may feel strong emotions like anger, sadness, grief, joy, or serenity, or you may feel very little. It can take practice to become familiar with our body sensations and the emotions that they evoke. This is just a first step.

Continue to observe the sensation and the emotions that you experience for a few more minutes. Do the feelings stay the same? Do they shift or change to other emotions? Are they pleasant or unpleasant? Do you feel comfortable paying attention to the feelings or experience the desire to shift your focus? Once you've spent about five minutes getting familiar with these sensations and any feelings that arise, take a break. Then reflect on the questions above and your experience while doing this exercise. Did you learn anything new about yourself?

The exercise of attuning to your bodily sensations and emotions is very useful for discovering where you hold emotional energy and experience in your body. This energy and emotion may be related to the present moment, or a vestige of past experience. Once you gain familiarity with your bodily states and related emotions you will become more able to detect subtle shifts in your feeling states, and know when you are physiologically flooded and the limbic system has made effective communication difficult, if not impossible. That is your cue to take a break, practice intentional breathing, and regain your equilibrium rather than react.

Modulating the Release Valve

Bessel van der Kolk is a psychiatrist and leading expert on mind–body approaches in the treatment of trauma and post-traumatic stress disorder (PTSD). In his influential book, *The Body Keeps the Score: Brain, Mind and Body in the Healing of Trauma*, he discusses how traumatic and painful events and memories become stored in our bodies, sometimes so deeply that we have little, if any, conscious awareness of them (van der Kolk 2014). Many of my clients with trauma histories report being aware of some distant, foggy memory of a traumatic experience but have little recollection of the event itself. They are often surprised to learn that emotional information can be stored within the body and nervous system, often for decades.

How does this suppression of emotion relate to intentional breathing? Imagine that your mind and body are like a pressure cooker. You endure high levels of stress, day after day. Your SNS deals with the stress by working overtime, containing the built-up energy and increasing the pressure on the system. Like any pressure cooker, you have the capacity to hold a great deal of energy without leaking or blowing your top because, like the container of the cooker, your nervous system has become very adept at holding it in. It is an adaptive way of preventing a meltdown, even if it isn't sustainable in the long run.

The very nature of living as a pressure cooker means that you become less attuned to your body and its sensations. If you open the lid even just a little bit, you may run the risk of being flooded by the pain, muscle contraction, shortness of breath, gastric upset, anxiety, depression, or myriad other symptoms that have built up over time. When you keep the lid tightly closed, you also become adept at tuning out or failing to recognize the body's signals that inform you that you are wearing out or breaking down. In a sense, you become disembodied.

It is important to remember that intentional breathing and somatic experiencing can function like a release valve. Open the valve too quickly and you run the risk of being overwhelmed by intense emotional energy. It works the same way with your autonomic nervous system. If you rapidly shift your state from highly charged sympathetic arousal to deeply relaxed parasympathetic dominance, your system may become destabilized. Feelings of mild to intense anxiety and emotional upset may arise if you attempt to force a change too rapidly. In this case, more is not necessarily better. Instead, slow, tempered practice allows your brain, body, and mind to acclimate to a new state of relaxation and body awareness rather than trying to force it into a way of being that it may not be used to. This is why I suggest exploring bodily sensations slowly. Move too rapidly and the input may seem over-whelming at first, particularly if you have a life of "stuffing" unpleasant emotions or have little awareness of your somatic experience.

Emotional awareness and expression are key precursors to emotional intelligence (Goleman 2005) and good health (Mate 2011; Sternberg 2001). By understanding your feeling experience, you will become able to modulate it, choosing when, where, how, and with whom you express negative emotions like anger, aggression, anxiety, defen-siveness, or despair or positive feelings like love, joy, gratitude, hope, and contentment. The more attuned you are to your body and its feeling states, the more skilled you will become. It is a matter of consistent practice and a commitment to your wellbeing and to the bettering of your relationships.

11 | Appraising and Adjusting Your Mindset

There is nothing more important to true growth than realizing that you are not the voice of the mind – you are the one who hears it.

Michael A. Singer

Once you learn to calm your physiological stress response and become familiar with signs of emotional overwhelm, you create space for present awareness. This awareness allows you to observe your personal stories, emotions, and actions with greater clarity and understanding. It also creates the opportunity to appraise these narratives and mindsets and explore how they play out in your relationships.

Appraisal refers to the evaluation of the impact of a particular thought, feeling, behavior, or event on wellbeing. Psychologist Richard Lazarus proposed that the experience of psychological stress depends on how we appraise a situation. The more we appraise an event as stressful, the more we are likely to experience it as such (Lazarus & Folkman 1984; Folkman et al. 1986). Lazarus divided appraisal into two categories: primary and secondary. Primary appraisal involves the evaluation of what is at stake. For example, does a circumstance pose a threat to my wellbeing or the health and happiness of someone I love? Is my ego or self-esteem being challenged? Does this affect the bottom line of my organization? Secondary appraisal relates to the assessment of what we can do to increase benefit or reduce harm. It can directly shape how you cope with an event.

Coping refers to what you actively think or do when confronted with a demand that needs to be managed or changed. How you cope depends not only on your perception of the event but whether you believe you possess the capacity to change it. The more powerless you feel, the more likely you are to experience stress, and the less likely you may be to take effective action (Lazarus & Folkman 1984; Folkman et al. 1986). This occurs, in part, because physiological stress decreases the availability of cognitive resources.

The interdependence between stress, perception, and coping figures prominently in relationships. When under duress, you are more likely to appraise others negatively and react with aggression, withdrawal, criticism, and defensiveness. A study by Lazarus and colleagues illustrates this relationship between appraisal and coping skill (Folkman et al. 1986). Eighty-five married couples were interviewed once per month for six months. During the interview, each person was asked to discuss his or her most stressful encounter from the previous week. Responses were compiled and analyzed to examine each couple's appraisal strategy and coping style. The effectiveness of a couple's coping was directly related to their appraisal of the event. Married couples were less able to cope effectively when one or both members perceived an event as stressful. This suggests that the perception of a circumstance as stressful can undermine how effective we are at coping with it in the context of a relationship. This is one reason why it is important to become aware of your stress response, experience of flooding, emotional state, perceptions, and personal narratives. With that awareness you can choose more effective coping methods rather than falling into habitual or reactive patterns.

EXERCISE
Exploring Your Appraisal and Coping Style

Find a quiet place where you can sit for roughly 10–15 minutes without interruption. Take a few moments to practice the intentional breathing exercise in Chapter 9. Once you feel comfortable and relaxed, bring your attention to one challenging or demanding circumstance in your life – your bills, kids, job, parents, or spouse. Imagine that person or situation in as much detail as you can, including your thoughts, feelings, stories about the situation, and any sensations that you feel in your body. Then ask yourself the following questions. Take a few minutes to write down your responses:

What comes to mind when I think of this person or situation?

Do I feel physically or emotionally tense or uncomfortable?

Where do I experience sensations in my body?

Do I excessively ruminate or worry about this situation or person?

What is my story about this person or circumstance?

How does that story relate to any of my other personal stories?

How do I cope with this challenge?

Do I avoid the person or circumstance altogether or wish it would just go away?

Do I confront the problem head on and do my best to change things?

Do I feel able to change the situation or do I feel powerless or incompetent?

How do my feelings of being empowered or powerless relate to whether or not I experience this circumstance or person as stressful?

What did I learn from this exercise?

Stress is Inevitable, Distress is Optional

Demanding life circumstances are inevitable. Although you can't always control them, you can choose how to respond. You may deal with them or perpetuate them. In other words, you may choose to generate stress, reduce it, or end your experience of stress altogether.

Picture yourself driving down the street when the car next to you rapidly begins to switch lanes, nearly forcing you off the road. Immediately, your sympathetic nervous system (SNS) kicks into gear and you swerve to avoid an accident. You're now flooded with a cascade of stress hormones. Norepinephrine, adrenaline, and cortisol are surging through your body. Your heart is pounding and you may be sweating and feeling nauseated all in the blink of an eye. Once your physiological arousal recedes, you have one of two choices: you can move on or you can mentally re-enact the experience over and over again, perpetuating your stress.

In the first case, you might think to yourself, "Wow, that was close! I'm really lucky I didn't get hit or someone didn't get hurt!" and leave it at that. Or you may launch into a rant, yell, swear, or try to catch up to the offending driver and give him a piece of your mind. You may even decide to drive excessively defensively to thwart other bad drivers who might potentially harm you. Depending on your coping style, you may obsess about the event all day, get upset about it again driving home, and recount the story to your spouse or friend and go to bed even more furious. That one, five-second event just became a day's worth of physiological and psychological stress. Just imagine the effect that that coping style, or something like it, might have on your stress level and health, not to mention your relationships.

As we examined in Chapter 3, prolonged exposure to stress, whether real or self-generated, adds up. It can lead to psychological burnout and physiological depletion, exhaustion, inflammation, illness, infertility, osteoporosis, heart disease, gastrointestinal illness, and more. Stress literally becomes stored in your tissues. This is why your appraisal of life events and your coping strategy is essential to your wellbeing. You not only have the ability to generate suffering, but you also possess the capacity to select healthy methods of coping.

Chanie Gorkin, an eleventh grade student from Brooklyn, New York wrote a poem that brilliantly illustrates this point. It provides a wonderful example of how appraisal impacts our perception of events even when the content remains the same. Read the poem from top to bottom. Then read the same words from bottom to top.

The Worst Day Ever?
By Chanie Gorkin

Today was the absolute worst day ever

And don't try to convince me that

There's something good in every day

Because, when you take a closer look,

This world is a pretty evil place.

Even if

Some goodness does shine through once in a while

Satisfaction and happiness don't last

And it's not true that

It's all in the mind and heart

Because

True happiness can be obtained

Only if one's surroundings are good

It's not true that good exists

I'm sure you can agree that

The reality

Creates

My attitude

It's all beyond my control

And you'll never in a million years hear me say that

Today was a good day

Can you think of examples of ways in which your appraisal of your circumstances may negatively impact your life? Are there situations that you might appraise differently if you were able to consider them from an alternative point of view?

Skewed Appraisal: The Role of Attribution Bias

Your appraisal of events is often directly linked to your personal story. If you believe that the world is a dark, scary place, you are likely to interpret even benign events as dangerous. To quote Abraham Maslow, the American psychologist best known for creating his hierarchy of needs, "If all you have is a hammer, everything looks like a nail" (1966, p. 15).

Remember Joel who we first met in Chapter 4. Joel's personal narrative involved a fervent belief that no one liked him. He appraised everything from his professional stagnation to poor family relationships as being due to the fact that he did not fit in. This is called confirmation bias: the tendency to search for, interpret, and recall events that confirm your beliefs and stories while discounting or avoiding data that is inconsistent with these views (Nickerson 1998). Your personal narratives are often laden with bias, which is why you need to remain mindful of them and observe their impact on your perceptions and behavior.

Attribution bias is another form of misinterpretation that is shaped by your personal stories. This bias refers to a systematic error that you make when interpreting and judging the behavior of others (Heider 1958; Weiner 1992). Although there are various forms of attribution, causal attribution biases are particularly important in the context of relationships. Causal attributions involve judgments that an individual's behavior is due to internal factors (temperament, disposition, intention, etc.) or external circumstances (e.g. the weather, mechanical failure). The tendency to attribute behavior to internal or dispositional factors leads you to focus on the person rather than the context, making you more likely to assign blame rather than evaluate the circumstances objectively (Weiner 1992, 1995).

Take Joel, for example. Imagine he is sitting at his desk at work when a female colleague walks by and does not say hello. Given Joel's story that no one likes him, he is inclined to blame her neutral behavior on dispositional factors ("she's mean," "she doesn't like men," "she thinks that she's special") rather than considering external causes (her car broke down or she just had an argument with her partner, or she's busy and preoccupied thinking about a project). From this frame of reference, Joel builds up a treasure trove of negative experience and an even more elaborate personal story of being disliked and rejected. Given his mindset, he is more likely to respond to his colleague with hostility or contempt not only in the moment but in future interactions. His story strongly influences his perceptions, emotions, and behavior.

Attribution theorist and psychologist Harold Kelly and others have conducted considerable research into the mechanisms of attribution bias. They discovered that individuals are more likely to make inaccurate or hasty attributions regarding another's behavior when under duress (Kelly 1974). In other words, you are more likely to make errors in judgment and revert to your negative personal stories when you are feeling stressed (Hammond 1999). Stress limits our capacity to think mindfully. As you've seen with Joel, distorted attributions lead to inaccurate assumptions, poor coping behavior, and poor relationship quality. This is why getting a handle on chronic stress and becoming aware of your thoughts, emotions, stories, and sensations can reduce your reactivity and increase your ability to cope effectively with the challenges and demands of daily living.

Reappraisal: A Tool for Challenging Distorted Appraisals and Attributions

Language is powerful. There is a direct correlation between what you think, the words you use, and the life you have. If you want to change your life, change your story.

Barbara Stanny

When you fill your mind with past hurts and future fears, you compromise your ability to cope with the realities of the present. When you calm your nervous system using intentional breathing, you create space to examine your assumptions, appraisals, and attributions. Philosopher and psychologist William James once said, "The greatest weapon against stress is our ability to choose one thought over another." He was right. You possess the capacity to reappraise your thoughts and choose new responses, and can change your experience by altering your relationship to it. This is much easier to accomplish when you are in a relaxed state.

The Drama Experiment

Years ago, while in the midst of a difficult stretch, my friend Matt gave me some of the best advice I've ever received. He said, "Grace, you need a drama-free diet." At first, I wasn't sure what to make of that. I wasn't a drama queen and did my utmost to maintain a private life and avoid gossip. If anything, I was drama avoidant. So, what did it mean to live a drama-free life? Was I getting sucked into the theatrics of others? Was I so busy trying to be a good daughter, friend, colleague, and human being that I was undermining my happiness? Did it involve being more mindful in relationships? If so, how?

A few years later, I was editor-in-chief of a research journal – a position that required a great deal of skill, not to mention a thick skin. It is never fun to inform an author that her manuscript isn't acceptable for publication, or to receive angry, sometimes hurtful emails in return. This was fertile ground for a drama-free experiment. Personal attacks, whether on a screen or face-to-face, can trigger the same physiological reaction as an in-person confrontation. You become flooded. Your heart races or pounds, maybe your face flushes, or you start to shake or perspire. Your first coping strategy is often to attack/retaliate, defend, or avoid depending on which seems the most likely to obtain the desired result. Once that decision has been made, that's your story and you're sticking to it. At least, that is what happens when we fall prey to stress reactivity and any negative personal story we may be carrying. But there is another option.

Once I'd committed myself to a drama-free diet I became more sensitized to the idea of drama and began to look for it. It wasn't too difficult to find. Drama is embedded in personal stories. In these narratives, we are often cast as the victim, villain, or hero. Like the actors in a play, we use these roles to make sense of our interactions with others. Without awareness, the actor and the story are nearly inseparable.

The first order of business in my drama-free experiment was to create space between myself and the situation. Immediately after reading an unpleasant email, I made a pact with myself to take my dog for a walk. Here I found myself ruminating, alternating between anger, hurt, and defensiveness. Inevitably, this process would bring up a story. Once I recognized the story, I paid attention to it. Often, I found myself thinking that I was "supposed" to please others. By saying no, I had become the villain; a role that was in direct conflict with being a pleaser. I experienced this discrepancy between my old story, and the new drama-free one that I was rewriting as a major source of stress. I explored the physical and emotional sensations that arose as I sat with the story. The fear of not pleasing others felt like a weight on my heart. The drama evoked a knot in my stomach. My first instinct was to escape the lousy feelings by being the "pleaser" and appeasing the author of the email. That wouldn't work. I needed to figure out how to cope with this information and formulate an effective response.

When we react immediately to drama or other forms of emotional or physical provocation, we often resort to one or all of what psychologist John Gottman (1999) calls the Four Horsemen of the Apocalypse – attack or criticize, respond with contempt, defend, or stonewall (avoid communication). Hostile attacks, be they electronic or otherwise, can cause the same physiological flooding that in-person disagreements do. As we learned from the work of Gottman and others, when flooded, we are likely to be mindless and reactive, rather than thoughtful and responsive.

My drama-free experiment revealed that taking space between my appraisal and reaction yielded a lot of useful information. I learned that my experience of drama was so unpleasant that my first instinct was to end it immediately. Had I followed that urge, I would have found myself apologizing and backpedaling, neither of which would have been appropriate. Instead, I made a commitment to myself to take 24 hours before responding to an upsetting email. Once that time had passed, it was much easier to read the message again, empathize with the author's feelings of disappointment, and address the content of the email directly, rather than taking offense or reacting negatively. In this case, allowing myself the time to calm down, recognize the stories that were triggered in me, and reappraise the situation allowed me to empathize with the author and to craft a thoughtful response, rather than reacting with hostility or ignoring the author's bid to be heard and understood.

The Drama Decision Tree

This drama experiment led to the creation of a simple drama decision tree (Figure 11.1). The tree includes two major branches: intervention or reaction. When confronted with a difficult interaction you tend to experience an immediate reaction. That reaction may include a rash judgment about the person or situation that is colored by your stories and projections. For example, a harsh, combative email arrives. I experience the message as hurtful and I am angry. I make the attribution that the email's author is hostile and unprofessional. My immediate (and thoughtless) reaction would be to fire back with a similarly toned message. The result? I have just become an actor in a dramatic play.

The other branch of the drama decision tree involves taking what I call a purposeful pause, which will be covered in greater detail in Chapter 12. When you take a purposeful pause, you make a conscious commitment to create space between an unpleasant interaction and your response, rather than rushing in full of limbic overload and adrenaline and doing something you may regret. As part of that pause, you can practice intentional breathing to reduce the stress response and cultivate present-focused awareness, experience emotions that arise, and make a conscious decision to appraise the situation as accurately as possible and respond from a place of calm rather than reactivity. Here you allow the brain and body to work coherently, rather than engaging in stress-driven "bottom-up" processing, where the emotion centers of the brain dominate. This allows you to check your drama meter, recalibrate your physiology, and reappraise the situation from a place of equanimity rather than defensiveness or aggression.

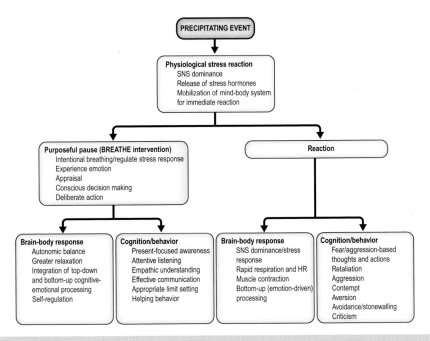

Figure 11.1

Drama Decision Tree

Reappraisal can be challenging, particularly when it conflicts with your personal stories. This is just as true at home as in the workplace. In my courses and workshops, participants often speak of the "Bully Boss," a supervisor who either willfully or passively makes life miserable by exerting his or her authority and making inappropriate requests. These circumstances can be particularly stressful and difficult when we feel helpless or powerless, or that our jobs may be in jeopardy. I once worked for a supervisor who frequently telephoned staff about non-urgent matters on evenings and weekends. These calls often involved allaying his stress and anxiety around workplace issues. Being that he was my supervisor, I initially felt caught between a rock and a hard place. My personal story of being a pleaser dictated that I be available and respond to his requests. On the flip side, I also had a drama-free policy, not to mention the fact that my health, sanity, and relationships depended on my ability to exercise personal boundaries around work. It felt like a no-win situation.

At first, I would answer his calls on a Saturday and spend an hour on the phone talking about work. This would be followed by a sleepless night ruminating about my job and feeling miserable the next day. Even though I was acutely aware of the consequences, I continued to answer the phone. Over time, I became angry and resentful. I switched to a second reaction – stonewalling. I blew off the calls altogether, fully knowing that I would hear about it the following day. Even though it seemed like a better alternative, I was still being emotionally reactive rather than mindfully responsive.

After several months of this, I became thoroughly fed up. The calls weren't stopping and my coping strategy was failing miserably. Out of desperation, I decided to try something different. I began to notice my reaction when the phone would ring. Inevitably, my breath became shallow and rapid, my chest tightened, and my stomach clenched. The story of failing to be available and disappointing my boss, family, and friends resonated in my head. The appraisal that my supervisor was an insensitive, disrespectful so-and-so led me to want to give him a piece of my mind. But I couldn't.

Instead, I allowed the call to go to voicemail. I took time to breathe intentionally until I no longer felt the physical and emotional cues of overwhelm. From that place of awareness and presence, it occurred to me that my supervisor was alone and unhappy. Like me, he was also feeling anxious and unsettled about work. From that vantage point, I discovered an empathic coping response that left me feeling empowered rather than victimized. The following day, I met my boss, acknowledged his voicemail and his distress, and made it clear that I was not able to discuss non-urgent work issues during off hours. I set clear boundaries and limits around my personal time. It wasn't easy. What I did discover was that it was easier to clearly articulate my limits, and work with my boss toward a solution when I approached him from a place of equanimity and empathic understanding rather than frustration. The calls stopped immediately. I was no longer participating in the drama. Had I stuck with my angry, defensive, or stonewalling posture, that likely would not have happened.

This is just one of the many circumstances that inspired the seven skills of BREATHE. Whether at home, work, or anywhere else in life, it is important to create space to evaluate your circumstances and the people in your life as clearly as possible. This can't be done when stress is chronically raging out of control. Once you take responsibility for managing stress, you can begin to recognize its impact on your thoughts, emotions, sensations, and behavior. From this place of awareness, you are more apt to accurately recognize your contribution to the dynamics you share with others. This empowers you to make decisions from a place of calm rather than reactivity, and is the key to building healthy and sustainable relationships.

Turning Stressors into Opportunities

When you begin to recognize sensations of stress or notice the impulse to fight, flee, or freeze, you've moved into what I call the discomfort zone. This zone is the first sign that you are moving from autopilot to awareness. This allows you to use the physiological and emotional cues that we explored in previous chapters as opportunities for self-understanding and growth. When you observe your reactions closely, there is a very good chance that you will detect a pattern. You may notice a tendency to feel certain emotions in specific regions of your body. You may also become familiar with your stories and recognize which ones pop up in the face of certain interpersonal challenges. As you may have already discovered, intentional breathing can get you back to solid footing before you let these sensations, thoughts, feelings, and emotions dictate your behavior.

EXERCISE
Working with Your Stories

Most of the time, when confronted with interpersonal conflict or other stressors, we avoid, resist, confront, or catastrophize. This reaction is habitual. You may not even be aware of it at first. It's not that this response is bad. It is a coping mechanism that you developed early in life, and with repeated practice it became second nature. However, in the present, it may be unskillful or potentially destructive to your personal and professional relationships. Although it can be extremely uncomfortable, your discomfort zone creates the opportunity to reappraise your circumstances and ask yourself, "Does the situation trigger a negative or unhelpful personal story?"

Sometimes identifying a story is easier than you think. Take a moment to recall a very recent stressful experience that you shared with another person. Try to remember the event as vividly as you can.

Now write down your response to the following questions.

What personal story or belief did I tell myself during this experience? (e.g. "I am a good person," "I am a failure," "I make everyone happy at my own expense," "I should be nice no matter what," "Nobody likes me," "I need to be right.")

Is that story true for me now?

Do I want to continue living this story?

Questioning your story can and often does initiate a process of reappraisal. Reappraisal involves questioning your attitudes, attributions, and your story's role in shaping them. From here, you may view situations differently and find alternative responses.

Years ago, while completing my clinical internship at the School of Medicine at the University of Washington, I had a very challenging client. No matter how hard I attempted to listen and respond to her needs, she appeared consistently unhappy. Having never been in that situation, I alternated between feeling disillusioned and incompetent. I frequently found myself fighting the desire to quit and avoid the grief of feeling inept. What's worse, I also became gripped by imposter syndrome.

Imposter syndrome refers to a deeply held belief that you've been given an opportunity for which you're not qualified. Yolanda's story in Chapter 4 is a good example of this. It's that gnawing sense of unease when you feel over your head and don't want to be found out. It feels awful! Instead of confronting the fear, it feels easier to bury your head in the sand and hope it will go away. Imposter syndrome is very common among first-year graduate, medical and law students. It tends to arise when we accept opportunities that push us beyond our comfort zone, or when one or more personal stories of incompetence, unworthiness, or fear of failure are triggered. In this case, I began to dread our sessions. I constantly worried that I was going to fail no matter how hard I prepared. It took the joy out of the job and left me performing at less than my best.

Several weeks into our work together, I knew that I had to either change course or refer my client to someone else. I decided to take a step back and assess which piece of the imposter story was true for me and which piece of my story was being fueled by fear and anxiety. It didn't take long before I realized that my client's unhappiness was due, in part, to my inability to clearly define the parameters and goals of our work together. They were also the result of the client's inability to articulate her needs and aspirations. From here, I was able to take responsibility for my part in our dynamic and realistically assess what was happening and why. Instead of succumbing to my personal imposter story and letting my stress physiology and emotional angst override mindful decision-making, I learned to openly articulate what was needed for our sessions to progress. Reappraisal gave me a realistic picture of what was playing out and allowed me to respond with clarity, calm, and skill in an otherwise stressful situation. From this, I learned that events that I perceived as stressful and challenging were often a catalyst for growth and that harnessing that potential transformed stressful circumstances into stories of empowerment and success. Stress is inevitable. Suffering is optional.

EXERCISE
Reappraising Your Story

Take some time to write down three situations or people in your life that you are struggling with or that you experience as stressful. It can be a situation or person at work or involve family or friends, your neighbors, or even your dog or cat. Just think of three things that are driving you nuts and write them down. Don't censor yourself. There is no right or wrong answer. Just write.

Once you've identified three situations, pick one and write down your responses to the following questions.

1. How much does this situation/person bother me?

   1 = not at all; 2 = a little bit; 3 = somewhat; 4 = quite a bit; 5 = very much

2. What personal story am I telling myself around this situation/person?

3. What is my typical response to the situation/person?

4. Do I have the ability to change the circumstances?

5. Can I think about this situation/person differently?

6. Can I react to this situation/person differently? If so, how?

7. Am I willing to change my thoughts about the situation?

8. Am I willing to change my feelings about the situation?

9. Am I willing to respond to the situation differently?

10. How much of this situation is about me? How much is about the other person?

11. How much of this is my responsibility to change?

Now look back at your responses and see whether you can detect any themes in your stories. What do these themes or stories tell you about yourself? If you'd like, try the exercise again for the other two situations that you identified.

You Are Not Your Story

This chapter began with a favorite quote from Michael A. Singer, bestselling author of two wonderful books, *The Untethered Soul* and *The Surrender Experiment*. Singer writes, "There is nothing more important to true growth than realizing that you are not the voice of the mind – you are the one who hears it" (Singer 2007, p. 5). In other words, our stories are just that – stories.

The most effective strategy for working with your personal narratives or readjusting your mindset is to observe your stories objectively, and to refrain from getting too attached to them. Most importantly, it is essential to remember that you are not your story and that it does not define you. Your stories are one of myriad thoughts that go streaming through your mental database nonstop. It is part of being human. As Michael Singer notes, "If you watch [the mind] objectively, you will come to see that much of what the voice says is meaningless. Most of the talking is just a waste of time and energy. The truth is most of life will unfold in accordance with forces far outside your control, regardless of what your mind says about it," (Singer 2007, p. 10).

So why do we spend so much time obsessing about things that we can't influence? Singer suggests that persistent fluctuations of the mind are, in part, a mechanism that we use to give ourselves a false sense of control. If we think about life enough, we may be able to change the outcome. Well, not really, but we think that we can. According to Singer, "You will come to see that the mind talks all the time because you gave it a job to do. You use it as a protection mechanism, a form of defense. Ultimately, it makes you feel more secure. As long as that's what you want, you will be forced to constantly use your mind to buffer yourself from life, instead of living it" (Singer 2007, p. 10). As we've seen from Joel's example, a harsh, critical, fearful voice does not protect you from what you fear most. In fact, it creates it. It clouds your lens of perception and frames the world in a way that can potentially cause you, and those around you, suffering. "True personal growth," says Singer "is about transcending that part of you that is not okay and needs protection. This is done by constantly remembering that you are the one inside that notices the voice talking…To be aware that you are watching the voice talk is to stand on the threshold of a fantastic inner journey. If used properly, the same mental voice that has been a source of worry, distraction, and general neurosis can become the launching ground for true spiritual awakening. Come to know the one who watches the voice, and you will come to know one of the great mysteries of creation" (Singer 2007, p. 13).

Rewriting Your Story

In my experience teaching the seven skills of BREATHE in courses and workshops, I've observed an interesting phenomenon. Some participants readily dive into exploring their personal narratives, while others resist. These "resisters" often comment that they feel uncomfortable writing down a story that they are working to change or that is no longer true for them. Instead, they choose to write an "emergent story" – one that explores the person they'd like to become rather than the story that was written for them. This is where we are heading next.

Personal stories reflect a mindset. A mindset refers to a set of ideas, assumptions, or philosophies held by an individual, group, or institution that shape thoughts, feelings, and actions (Dweck 2007). It is based on the values that we hold about ourselves and the world in which we live. For example, if, like Joel, you have a mindset that the world and the people in it are hostile, unwelcoming, or judgmental, your response will reflect this belief.

In rethinking who you are and the relationships you would like to manifest, it is important not only to be aware of your stories but also the values that they reflect. Sometimes these values and stories are not in alignment. Rather than getting stuck in this discrepancy, you can use this misalignment to examine what matters to you and write a new story. Not everyone will feel as though his or her values and stories are misaligned, however; some will observe a disconnect between who we aspire to be, the relationships we hope to create, and the stories that we tell ourselves. Wherever you land on this continuum, observe your responses and reactions from a place of exploration rather than indicting yourself for what you don't like. Remember that it took years for these stories to evolve and it will likely take time for them to be rewritten. This work is a process far more than it is a destination.

> **EXERCISE**
> **Exploring Your Values**
>
> Begin with a few minutes of intentional breathing to bring yourself into the present moment.
>
> Now take a look at the list below and circle your top 10 values (Table 11.1). This list is not exhaustive.
>
> If something is missing please feel free to add it.
>
> Once you've identified your top 10 spend a few moments identifying your top three most preferred values.

TABLE 11.1 List of Values		
Acceptance	Ethics	Mental sharpness
Accountability	Excellence	Mindfulness
Achievement	Fairness	Nature
Adaptability	Family	Open communication
Ambition	Financial stability	Openness
Artistry	Forgiveness	Patience
Attitude	Friendships	Perseverance
Awareness	Freedom	Personal fulfillment
Balance (home/work)	Fun	Personal growth
Beauty	Future generations	Physical achievement
Being the best	Generosity	Physical strength
Caring	Gratitude	Power
Coaching/mentoring	Happiness	Professional growth
Commitment	Hard work	Recognition
Community involvement	Harmony	Reliability
Compassion	Health	Resourcefulness
Competence	Helping others	Respect
Conflict resolution	Honesty	Responsibility
Continuous learning	Humility	Risk-taking
Cooperation	Humor/fun	Safety
Courage	Inclusion	Self-discipline
Creating peace	Independence	Social justice
Creativity	Ingenuity	Spiritual growth
Curiosity	Integrity	Strength
Dialogue	Interdependence	Success
Discipline	Initiative	Teamwork
Discovery	Innovation	Trust
Ease with uncertainty	Intuition	Vision
Enthusiasm	Job security	Wealth
Entrepreneurial	Leadership	Well-being
Environmental sustainability	Learning	Willpower
	Listening	Wisdom
Equality	Making a difference	World peace

Once you have identified your top three, pick one and write your responses to the following questions. As you explore these answers, remember that the purpose of the exercise isn't to evaluate how "good" you are at living up to these values and aspirations.

This exercise is intended to get you in touch with your deepest values and how they may, or may not influence your current story, decisions, and actions.

1. Why is this value most important to you?

2. How does this value affect how you treat yourself?

3. How does this value affect how you treat others?

4. How does this value guide your decision-making?

5. Is this value reflected in your personal story? How?

6. Is this your value or one that was given to you by someone else?

One of the most powerful ways to change your personal story is to rewrite it. As you write, you may discover that you're already living it, or you may learn that your current mindset may be standing in the way of the person you'd like to be. What matters most is the insight you gain from the experience of writing your story and not whether or not you are currently living it.

EXERCISE
Rewriting Your Story

Take some time in a quiet place to reflect on the story that you would like to write for yourself. It could be a story of who you are, who you would like to become, who you would like to be in relationships with family, close friends, your spouse or partner, or your colleagues. If you find that it seems like a big undertaking to rewrite or revise your story, consider looking at your responses to the values exercise above and see if you can rewrite your story in a way that reflects your top values.

12 | Taking a Purposeful Pause

Take rest, a field that has rested gives a bountiful crop.

Ovid

Speed is irrelevant if you're traveling in the wrong direction.

Mahatma Gandhi

Years ago, while studying film and television scoring at UCLA, I made an interesting discovery. As a new student, I believed that successful music composers filled the space with as many notes as possible, and that the goal of creating great music was to cleverly use as many orchestral instruments as your imagination would allow. Then one day I was asked to compose music for a film clip using only a harmonica, flute, bassoon, and stand-up bass. I was dumbfounded. No matter how hard I tried, I could not find a way to harmoniously arrange these four instruments together. Each attempt sounded like fingernails scratching across a chalkboard to me. I was dismayed. I decided to step back and reassess my strategy of filling the page with notes and spent the next two days listening to the works of several of my favorite composers including Wolfgang Amadeus Mozart and James Horner. What I discovered shocked me. Their compositions had as much (if not more) to do with the spaces between the notes as the notes themselves. The magic seemed to occur in the moments of pause when I held my breath in anticipation of a resolution, or felt my body soften as stillness washed over me. The same principle applies to life.

For better or worse, "work hard play hard" is the ethos of our competitive culture. This is particularly the case when fear and stress are high. Research is beginning to demonstrate that sleep and taking breaks are key for maintaining health and boosting learning, creativity, and productivity (Binnewies, Sonnetag & Mozja 2010; Gottselig et al. 2004; Oppezzo & Schwartz 2014; Sonnetag 2003; Sonnetag & Fritz 2006, 2007; Stickgold et al. 2001). Paradoxically, doing less may inevitably result in getting more done.

This need to take time to restore is rooted in our physiology (Benson, Beary, & Carol 1974). As we've discovered, systems designed for rest and repair are wired into our brains and bodies. But many of us try to supplant restoration with caffeine, sugar, and the rush of adrenaline that we get by exercising hard or living on the edge. This type of high-intensity lifestyle can, and often does, lead to physical and emotional burnout.

Burnout is the result of prolonged exposure to interpersonal and emotional job stress. Most of what we know about burnout comes from research in the workplace (e.g. Ahola et al. 2014; Bakker & Costa 2014; Innanen, Tolvanen, & Salmela-Aro 2014; Llorens-Gumbau & Salanova-Soria 2014). As it relates to job performance, burnout is usually defined by several factors including physical and psychological exhaustion, cynicism, detachment from the job, a sense of ineffectiveness and poor work performance. In her influential book, *The Balance Within: The Science Connecting Health and Emotions* (2001), internationally recognized expert in the science of mind-body interactions, stress and wellness, Dr. Esther Sternberg points to the significant toll that burnout takes on those in helping professions including the inability to respond to even slight stressors. This depletion of human resources may be one reason why burnout is a recognized phenomenon in most employment sectors. A review of the scientific evidence suggests that employee burnout can have catastrophic effects on job performance, including absenteeism, decreased job satisfaction, reduced commitment, and job turnover. What's more, burnout can have a spillover effect into your personal world, leading to an overall decreased quality of life (Haslach, Schaufelt, & Leiter 2001).

As you can imagine, high levels of stress, excessive work demands, and social and economic pressures make burnout highly prevalent. This may be because workers are reluctant to take time off to rest and recuperate. According to a 2015 article published in *Fortune Magazine*, American workers do not come close to utilizing their paid vacation days (Fisher 2015). In the survey, 72% of senior managers and 56% of employees said that they would not use more vacation time than they currently do even if their companies offered unlimited paid vacation. According to Diane Domeyer, executive director of the Creative Group, the company that conducted the survey, people find the idea of being away from work stressful because of the amount of work that they fear will pile up in their absence. People also save vacation time in case they may need time off because of illness or a family emergency. No matter how you look at it, in spite of emerging research that suggests that taking time off can increase learning and productivity and improve life satisfaction, many are unwilling or unable to make sufficient time to rest.

Sabine Sonnetag, professor of work and organizational psychology at the University of Konstanz in Germany, studies the balance between rest and recovery and job performance. Sonnetag and her colleagues have found that taking time off has positive effects on engagement and proactive behaviors at work, like taking the initiative to begin a project (Sonnetag 2003). In a study of 147 employees from six organizations who responded to a questionnaire about their job characteristics, engagement, and proactive behavior, Sonnetag found that taking a break for even a few minutes was associated with increased engagement and proactive behavior. What's more, this relationship was found even after accounting for an individual's natural tendency to be engaged and proactive (Sonnetag 2003).

In another study, Sonnetag and colleagues found that taking a break may be even more important after extremely stressful work days. She asked 133 adults to complete weekly questionnaires over four weeks about their work and rest experience. Employees who took time to recover from work stress showed greater task performance, perceived effort, personal initiative, and "organizational citizenship," suggesting that taking time off is beneficial both for individuals and the organizations where they work (Binnewies et al. 2010). This doesn't just apply to short breaks. In a study of 221 university employees who completed a survey about their health complaints, burnout level, task performance, and effort on the job, positive changes in wellbeing and increased expenditure of effort were reported following an extended vacation (Sonnetag & Fritz 2006). Collectively, these studies concur that time off, whether a few hours or a prolonged vacation, benefits not only individual employees but their organizations as well.

The lack of rest in modern society seems to be reaching a crisis point according to psychologist James Mass and his colleagues in, *Power Sleep: The Revolutionary Program That Prepares Your Mind for Peak Performance* (Maas et al. 1999). Here they note, "If you're getting less than eight hours' sleep each night, including weekends, or if you fall asleep instantly, or need an alarm clock to wake up, consider yourself one of the millions of chronically sleep-deprived people – perhaps blissfully ignorant of how sleepy and ineffective you are, or how dynamic you could be with adequate sleep," (Maas et al. 1999, p. 5). Moreover, "According to sleep experts, if you want to be fully alert, in a good mood, mentally sharp, creative, and energetic all day long, you might need to spend at least one third of your life sleeping," (Maas et al. 1999, p. 6).

In addition to demonstrating personal and professional benefits and improving your health and wellbeing, neuroscientific evidence points to sleep as important for cognitive functioning (Gottselig et al. 2004; Stickgold et al. 2001). Sleep aids learning and memory, including the development of problem-solving skills and procedural learning. Some of this information processing occurs during the rapid eye movement (REM) phase of sleep (Stickgold et al. 2001). REM sleep, a deep stage of rest in which dreams occur, is also associated with the processing of emotional memories (Groch et al. 2013). Conversely, the absence of good quality sleep is linked to a wide range of psychiatric disorders including major depression, anxiety, and post-traumatic stress disorder (Krystal 2012). By and large, the research shows that sleep is essential for cognitive performance and psychological health. In the absence of sufficient, quality rest, we are less likely to process information accurately or effectively, or engage others mindfully or successfully.

Taking a Pause in Relationship

Taking time off isn't just about getting enough rest. The degree to which you rest and care for your physical and psychological wellbeing can also impact your behavior in relationships. Western culture places value on rapid responding, fast and efficient problem solving, being on the attack, and getting the job done. These values shape our style of relating to others. We plow into conversations more concerned with getting our point across, winning, or being heard than listening and creating room for a deeper understanding of the other.

Indian spiritual teacher Sai Baba was a great proponent of silence and intentional speech. He is quoted as saying, "Before you speak, ask yourself, 'Is it kind, is it necessary, is it true, does it improve on the silence?'" As a psychologist, researcher, and intent observer of interpersonal dynamics, I found this quote particularly striking. In my observation, a great deal of human communication is marked by a need to be heard, rather than to listen. However, attention to and awareness of the communication process, and our role in it, is a hallmark of mindful interaction. Although it may seem as though communicating mindfully may be a relatively simple task, pausing to create space for others to be heard can be remarkably difficult, particularly if we feel excited, threatened, triggered, or defensive, or perceive silence as a sign of weakness or indecision.

When it comes to communication, silence can be golden. A cacophony can be downright unpleasant, not to mention ineffectual. Conversations are like building a fire. If we haphazardly dump as many logs as possible into a hearth without creating space for the air to circulate, the fire quickly dies. Likewise, if we bombard others with our thoughts without creating space for them in the conversation, they rapidly lose interest and we miss the opportunity to connect.

Many of us have been conditioned to believe that conversations are exercises in turn taking. Unfortunately, this strategy can also yield very unsatisfying results for both the speaker and the listener. While living in Massachusetts, I made a new friend who was very bright and engaging, and had a diverse set of skills and interests that I enjoyed hearing about. Early in getting to know each other, I observed that each time I would tell a story, he would respond by recounting a story of his own. While I was speaking, I could literally see his mind working on what he was about to say next. It didn't take long to realize that he wasn't really listening or taking in what I was saying – rather, it felt more like a tennis match in which ideas were being volleyed back and forth. When we were together, I could feel my body tensing up as I finished a sentence, and my heart sink when he immediately jumped in with a story of his own. I often felt unheard, unappreciated, and marginalized. When I commented on my experience, he respond-ed by saying, "Well, isn't that what I'm supposed to do … respond to your story with one of my own?" Given how much that dynamic undermined our ability to get to know each other and build a friendship, I'd say that the answer was no.

Good discussions aren't just about information exchange. They also provide oppor-tunities for listening, understanding, reflecting, and learning. When you concentrate on conversational turn taking more than listening or creating space for others to par-ticipate, you lose the capacity to be present because your mind is busy working on what to say next. This circumvents the opportunity to create meaningful connection.

Holding the Space

John Kabat-Zinn, creator of Mindfulness-Based Stress Reduction (MBSR), defines mind-fulness as "paying attention, in a particular way, on purpose, in the present moment, non-judgmentally" (1994, p. 4). In an interpersonal context, this means several things:

1. Setting an intention to pause and observe your habitual response tendencies.
2. Examining how your perceptions, personal stories, and communication patterns affect others.
3. Committing yourself to listening rather than immediately responding.
4. Taking the time to hear someone out rather than criticizing, passing judgment, problem-solving, or responding by telling your story.
5. Approaching communication from the stance of an impartial observer rather than an evaluator – meaning, not placing value judgments on yourself or others.
6. Knowing when you are physiologically stressed and flooded and making a com-mitment to take a step back to recalibrate before causing harm.

The task of mindful listening is to establish a safe zone of respectful silence where others can explore and express their thoughts and feelings. In other words, instead of filling the silence with notes or stuffing the hearth with logs, you pause, wait, and listen. This doesn't mean that you don't participate in the conversation – rather, you allow it to flow like a meandering river rather than diverting its course or damming the current with your own needs, agendas, or anxieties. This can be remarkably challenging if your tendency is to problem-solve, help out, or fix things.

Holding the space and listening to others can be especially difficult when you feel stressed, anxious, or overwhelmed, or are wrestling with emotions like fear and anger. Here, you may innately resort to habitual response patterns like jumping in or checking out. Taking a pause in these circumstances allows you to recognize when you are feeling flooded, and to observe your natural response tendencies. However, the skill of pausing takes practice.

EXERCISE
Holding the Space

Find a place where you will not be distracted or interrupted for about 5–10 minutes. Leave your mobile devices behind (preferably, turn them off). Once you are seated comfortably, sit upright, lengthen your spine while keeping your face, neck, and shoulders relaxed. Then close your eyes or turn your gaze downward to reduce distraction. Then sit silently and still for 3–5 minutes. Once you are done, explore the following questions.

How did it feel to sit and do nothing?

How did it feel to be in silence?

What physical sensations did you notice?

Did your experience of sensations, thoughts, or feelings change as time passed?

Did you feel the need to do something, think about something, run a story through your mind, create a list, problem-solve, plan an activity, or something else?

Did sitting and doing nothing in silence with no particular agenda feel comfortable or uncomfortable?

Remember that there are no right or wrong answers. You are gathering information about your experience.

If you were somewhere between mildly uncomfortable and jumping out of your skin, you're not alone. Most adults struggle to some degree with sitting still and doing nothing. Here's an example. Yoga classes typically end with a period of time called *savasana* – several minutes in which participants lie on their backs in "corpse pose." The idea is to remain still in a state of relaxation to allow yourself to assimilate the effects of your practice. Simple enough? Not exactly.

When I first began to practice yoga, *savasana* was incredibly difficult. In fact, I couldn't do it. No sooner did the class wind down for corpse pose than I bolted out the door. The thought of lying still in a quiet room was untenable. I could not understand how busy people could lie around and do nothing. So I left. Eventually I decided to give it a try. With consistent practice, I was able to lie still for several minutes, and even began to look forward to the uninterrupted silence. Now, as I observe students wrestle with five or so minutes of lying still, I see that corpse pose offers valuable information about our comfort in taking purposeful pauses, or making room for our experience. If you struggle to create space for yourself, there's a good chance that you confront the same discomfort when interacting with others. The good news is that with time and practice you can become skilled at taking purposeful pauses and allowing others to do the same.

Here is my favorite strategy for practicing taking a purposeful pause. Set your phone, watch, computer, or a clock to chime once per hour during the day (or more frequently if you'd like more practice). When you hear that chime, stop what you are doing for 60 seconds, then notice your reaction. Chances are, it will vary from one time to the next, but you will gain some interesting information about your comfort with taking a pause, and how that varies over time. On some days, you may discover that you're more at ease, while on others you may feel frustrated, irritable, angry, or unwilling to stop what you're doing. When the latter occurs, you may want to make note of your feelings, then pay particular attention to how you relate to others.

These pauses also afford you the opportunity to practice other BREATHE skills. Take a few, deep intentional breaths, notice your physical or emotional state, and see if there are any stories that are running through your mind. All of these tools increase your familiarity with yourself, and the ways in which you relate to others and your world. The more accustomed you are to creating that space, the easier it becomes to offer it to those around you.

Creating space between an event and your response is an invaluable skill when dealing with others. In stepping back and allowing time to evaluate your mindset and gain perspective, you create the opportunity to experience the situation and others differently. Instead of defaulting to your usual story, you may realize that your unpleasant colleague has a sick child, or your distracted friend just lost their dog. Rather than reacting, this space allows you to reappraise the event and create alternative hypotheses around it. From there, you can formulate a thoughtful, and perhaps more empathic, compassionate response.

Pausing and making room for reappraisal isn't always easy, particularly if you are used to taking charge and getting things done. It can also be challenging in circumstances like sitting in a meeting, a parent–teacher conference, or finding yourself in the midst of a disagreement with your child, partner, or co-worker when you may not have the opportunity to create physical distance or temporal space to reappraise the situation. This is when intentional breathing is your best friend, because it is a skill that can be used even in the midst of a stressful event. By slowing down your respiration you create space for your physiology to calm down. This allows you to sense where in your body you are holding emotion, and identify your feelings and the stories that have been triggered. Here you may discover that the issue is not worth the conflict, that you don't want to participate in the drama, or that a situation or relationship is not healthy. From that place of awareness, you can choose a mindful response.

One of the best strategies for bringing pauses into my life has been to make an appointment with myself. Nearly 20 years ago, I began to schedule workouts during my lunch hour, making sure that they appeared in my schedule like any other engagement. I discovered that when these events were on my calendar, I tended to prioritize them. Instead of interrupting the flow of my work or reducing my productivity, I observed that these midday workouts actually enhanced my functioning. Similarly, by setting my computer to chime each hour, I create a purposeful moment to check-in with myself and assess my physical, emotional, and mental state. From here, I can make informed decisions about my actions, rather than inadvertently projecting my mood or stories onto others.

13 | Humor: Life as Practice

Life is too important to be taken seriously.

Oscar Wilde

I have seen what a laugh can do. It can transform almost unbearable tears into something bearable, even hopeful.

Bob Hope

You may not be able to change a situation, but with humor you can change your attitude about it.

Allen Klein

I grew up in a perfectionistic household. This perfectionism was accompanied by what I call "the tyranny of the should." I "should" be doing this. It "should" look this way or that. I "should" have known better. *Should* is an intolerant taskmaster. Sadly, many of us suffer from disillusionment and despair because we've been led to believe that we are inadequate, unworthy, or have unsuccessful because we *should* be doing something differently. We anticipate that our lives *should* be unfolding according to some predetermined plan, but for social, economic, and other reasons, many of these plans may not have manifested or have fallen apart. We wrestle with the stories of who we *should* be, and how our lives *should* unfold. But life is far from perfect, which is why we need tools to navigate the reality of imperfect living.

One of the most powerful tools for addressing the *tyranny of the should* is humor. Humor allows you to laugh at yourself and your circumstances, rather than playing out your stories. It allows you to challenge the reality of your expectations, and embrace your foibles and learn from them, rather than punish yourself for making errors. After all, mistakes are inherently human, and without them you would likely not learn many valuable lessons. This is not to devalue the pain and disappointment that you encounter in life, but to suggest that there are circumstances in which you create additional suffering by being unduly hard on yourself, rather than cutting yourself some slack.

I first entered the world of mindfulness practice as a student of the Soto Zen tradition. I was introduced to lengthy meditation practices that involved sitting and staring at a blank wall for extended periods of time. Like many, I was determined to become an exceptional meditator. I assumed that with enough time and practice, I would nail it. I would be able to sit for endless periods of time looking like all of the serene people around me. But that wasn't happening. The longer I sat, the more uncomfortable I became. My knees hurt. My back hurt. My feet hurt. My neck and shoulders would scream at me. I wanted to meditate perfectly so much that I put myself through a tremendous amount of suffering. I even spent a few weeks at a Zen monastery, convinced that total immersion in the practice would do the trick. It didn't.

Don't get me wrong. My time at the monastery yielded a great deal of insight into the workings of my mind. One of those insights was that perfectionism was killing me.

When you think about it, perfectionism is like a hamster wheel – you run incessantly with the hope of achieving something, but you can never get there, and you won't jump off for fear of failure or mediocrity. You do the same thing time and again, expecting different results, which, according to the great Albert Einstein, is the definition of insanity. It is exhausting. Imperfection is the essence of being human. It is what motivates us to change what isn't working and to accept what we can't change. It makes living authentically possible.

The sad reality is that many of us spend a lifetime resisting our imperfection until we are hit with injury, illness, aging, or death. It took a bad hip fracture for me to realize the futility of running on the wheel in pursuit of the elusive moment when everything in my life would measure up to my litany of unrealistic *shoulds*. I discovered that everything was OK just as it was – messes and all. I also began to recognize that the attitude with which I approach life determines the quality of my experience and the stories that I tell. Just like Joel, Suzanne, Tal, and Yolanda, my life and experiences are shaped by my attitude. If I am intolerant of my imperfection, I suffer. If I believe that walking the path of mindfulness will be eternally blissful, I will be disappointed.

We suffer when we become attached to unrealistic or perfectionistic beliefs. We also suffer when we take ourselves and others too seriously, expecting that all will work out according to plan and we will emerge from life's roller coaster ride without any bumps and bruises. While it may seem difficult to approach life with a light heart when we are in the midst of what can seem like interminable stress, relationship strife, darkness, or despair, sometimes those experiences provide striking contrast to the moments of lightness and joy. In other words, without the darkness, we would be unable to see the stars.

The Power of Persistence

The Merriam-Webster Dictionary defines persistence as a characteristic that allows an individual to continue along a course of action even though it is difficult or opposed by others (2016). Our lives, relationships, and mindfulness practices most certainly require this quality, particularly when we encounter periods when it feels as though the magic is gone and the attraction has faded. It is at this precise moment that perseverance can be most difficult. Add new practices like intentional breathing, body awareness, appraisal of our thoughts, and taking pauses when we feel the urge to act, and we feel like giving up.

When I encounter periods of doubt and uncertainty they remind me of one summer in my childhood when I placed a caterpillar in a jar so that I could witness the process of metamorphosis. Even though I had no idea whether to expect a moth or a butterfly, I prayed hard that a monarch butterfly would emerge. Each day, I ran to the window in great anticipation of a beautiful butterfly. Each day, my heart sank when I was met by the same dull gray, fading cocoon. At some point, I began to wonder if the creature in the cocoon had died. It seemed silly to put so much hope in something that appeared dead and place my faith in a dream that seemed like wishful thinking. I debated throwing in the towel and emptying out the jar, but some glimmer of promise and the hope of witnessing something magical kept me coming back.

In the end, that persistence was rewarded. One morning I woke to find a newly transformed winged moth in the jar. It wasn't a monarch, but she was just as beautiful in her own way. Like giving birth, that period of long incubation seemed worth it once the moth unfolded her speckled wings. Had I tried to accelerate the hands of time, the miracle would have never occurred or she would not have fully formed. Had I given up and thrown the jar away, I'd have missed one of nature's most spectacular transformations. Faith and persistence kept me coming back.

Like the metamorphoses of moths and butterflies, periods of unplanned stasis come without a timeline. Even if we attempt to impose one, we can never truly predict if or when our desired outcome will occur. In these periods of unknowing, our task is to persevere. Some days we may white knuckle it, while, on other days, we may choose to surrender to whatever arises or engage in a flurry of activity. There is no ideal solution. What matters most is realizing that we have the ability to choose our response. Intentional breathing and the practices in previous chapters offer methods to be able to choose that response. Whatever choice you make, the most important task of all is to keep practicing creating space for wise decision-making to occur. Keep breathing. Remain aware of the messages that your body, mind, and stories are communicating to you. Listen to what emerges.

Living a mindful life is a difficult business. Like anything worth doing, it requires discipline, persistence, and determination. I've learned a great deal about determination from writing. The process of putting word to paper can be as painful as it is rewarding. Most writers will tell you that there are days, weeks, even months when the well of words runs dry. No matter how many hours you spend staring at the computer screen, nothing seems to express what you're hoping to convey. No amount of will, force, or begging will change it. The trick is to show up to work each and every day and write. Something. Anything. You may end up tossing it in the end, but you have made the attempt. Eventually, that persistence will pay off.

Likewise, you can show up time and time again to work on a relationship and find yourself falling flat on your face. Just as you can't control when the writing muse will appear, you can't change how people respond. You can only dedicate yourself to embodying integrity, perseverance, compassion, respect, self-awareness, and a commitment to be mindful in your interactions. Then pick yourself up, dust yourself off, and try again.

Facing the anxieties of uncertainty and change, you can always rely on your breath and your capacity to alter it in a way that best serves you. Intentional breathing empowers you to address those aspects of your life that seem beyond your control. It grounds you physically and mentally. It also allows you to observe the stories you tell and the sensations that you experience, and to learn from them.

Like your relationships and other events in your life, the practices in the BREATHE model may lose their allure. In the beginning, they may seem like a shiny object or the solution to your hectic, stressful schedule. But, as with all things, inevitably the novelty wears off. Then you are faced with the task of deciding whether or not your practice is worth your time and effort. Do you choose to commit even though the object may appear tarnished or worn? Will you remain steadfast even during the days, weeks, or months when it just doesn't seem to be working? Can you delay immediate gratification knowing that, like a tree sitting dormant, you may not see new buds for months? Sure you can. A new cycle of birth will occur in its own time. It all comes down to having the faith to persist.

Pitfalls to Persistence

One of the biggest mindsets that makes persistence difficult is the belief that growth will always feel good. A second is taking yourself too seriously. As a culture, we've been led to believe that growth *should* be positive. But like birth, the process of giving life to something new can be prolonged and painful. As a scientist, I've observed that human "growth" occurs in both a positive and a negative direction. In other words, you can grow in the direction that you expect (positive), or feel as though you are regressing (negative). It's all a matter of perspective. What may seem like a slide into a period of darkness or a reversal into old, unhealthy behavior patterns can also be the catalyst for change in the right direction.

You may notice that even in writing about growth I'm confined to language that imposes a dichotomous value judgment – positive/negative, slide down/rise up, right/wrong. We've been conditioned to think in either–or rather than both–and terms, and our perceptions reflect that. While you may not easily conjure up examples of "negative" growth, periods of stress, chaos, and even depression can often precede positive transformation. It all depends on how you appraise the situation.

Appraisal can be, and often is, biased by a belief that life *should* be easy, or that challenges *should* be navigated with grace and ease. You've probably been told that if you work hard enough, things will get "better" rather than stagnate or get worse. You may even have been led to believe that "good" (or good enough) relationships are those that flow smoothly with little conflict. Likewise, you may hold the expectation that the trajectory of a mindfulness practice like breath work, yoga, or meditation only improves over time. In my experience, the body and mind do become more flexible, and negotiating stress, disappointment, and challenge becomes easier with time and practice. Here is where both–and comes into play. You may find that you're more mindful sometimes and also increasingly more aware of your mindlessness. You may become more adept at reducing drama, increasing relaxation, and decreasing stress, but also more cognizant of how you undermine your ability to achieve your goals. In essence, your practice makes you both more attentive to *and* more aware of these dynamics.

The Gift of Humor

Sometimes it takes falling flat on your face to understand why humor is such an important part of life. Last year a couple of my friends and I decided to repair some rotting boards on my deck. This involved tearing up old planks to make space for the new ones. At one point, I was on my knees trying to pull up a decayed slat with all my might. Little did I know, my friend Karyn had just finished cutting into another panel next to me. When I attempted to use that board for leverage, it gave way sending me hurling face first into the jagged beams below. Searing pain tore from my left cheekbone to my forehead. The world was blurry, and I felt like a cartoon character with stars spinning around her head.

As I pushed my way up, I met Karyn's worried eyes. "Are you OK?" she whispered. "I think so," I replied. Then we both burst out laughing. We laughed so hard that it hurt – literally – and I thought my head was going to explode from the pain and the vibration of my laughter. In that moment, skinned, bloodied, and covered in sawdust, I realized that I'd just survived a pretty spectacular face plant.

One of the things that I love about yoga is that it is filled with metaphors for life. Several times each year, I teach what I call the "face plant" class. Although the objective is not to fall flat on your face, it requires you to flirt with your fears and learn to fall gracefully (and safely). The class includes a number of reflections on perfectionism, humor, and a sequence of preparatory postures that culminate in *bakasana*, or crow pose. Crow pose involves planting your hands into the floor with your shoulders above your wrists, engaging your core and hugging your inner thighs into your relatively straight upper arms. Then, if possible, your feet leave the floor, your hips rise into the air and your body hovers above the ground face down. Some crows take flight; others collapse in a heap –sometimes face first.

Crow pose was the first yogic arm balance that I set my sights on learning. I approached it with determined ferocity, convinced that with enough power and precision, I could take flight. I was wrong. Crow pose is as much about surrender as it is about strength and tenacity. The more I tried to force it, the more often I fell. Falling came with intense frustration. I was overcome with internal admonishments and feelings of failure. In time, however, I realized that crow pose has little to do with nailing the pose and everything to do with how you fall out of it. After all, in the grand scheme of the things, it's just a yoga pose. As is true for much of life, sometimes you soar and sometimes you crash. The highs-and-lows are simply constant reminders that we are, indeed, human. Falling is inevitable. What determines whether or not you suffer is how you get back up.

Research suggests that humor can serve a significant function in increasing our resiliency to stress (Abel 1998; Labott et al. 1990; Lefcourt & Martin 1986; Martin & Dobbin 1988). Humor and laughter are known to decrease the production of stress hormones, induce relaxation, stimulate circulation, improve respiration, and boost immunity (Brownell & Gardner 1988; Fry 1992; Lefcourt, Davidson-Katz, & Kuenemen 1990). Humor is also known to increase positive mood and be directly related to the use of positive reappraisal and problem-solving coping strategies (Abel 2002). In a study of college students self-identified as either having a high or low sense of humor, psychologist Millicent Abel found that those with a sense of humor appraised situations as less stressful and reported lower levels of anxiety than those with low humor, despite experiencing a similar number of daily problems. This, she suggests, supports the view that humor is associated with more effective appraisal and coping strategies, lower levels of negative emotion, less psychological distress, and reduced physiological arousal (Abel 2002).

In a review of the research on the benefits of humor, psychologist Rod Martin notes, "A sense of humor may enable individuals to cope more effectively with stress by allowing them to gain perspective and distance themselves from a stressful situation, enhancing their feelings of mastery and wellbeing in the face of adversity. Indeed, there is considerable experimental and correlational evidence for the stress moderating effects of humor … Individuals with a good sense of humor may cope more effectively with stress than other people do and, therefore, might also experience fewer of the adverse effects of stress on their physical health" (Martin 2002, p.217). In his review, Martin also discovered that humor serves an important social function: "Humorous individuals find it easier to attract friends and develop a rich social-support network and, therefore, gain well-established health benefits of social support" (Martin 2002, p. 219). From what we have learned about the importance of social bonds in developing and maintaining psychological health, it is also likely that those with strong social bonds tend to be happier overall.

Once you cease to strive for perfection and release the need for achievement, you can embrace the ups and downs of your mindfulness practice and relationships with a bit more lightness and ease. This opens the door for humor, levity, and feelings of acceptance and gratitude, all which foster social connection. It is an imperfect journey, but it is well worth the effort.

Smile
By Charlie Chaplin

Smile, though your heart is aching.

Smile, even though it's breaking.

When there are clouds in the sky,

you'll get by.

If you smile through your fear and sorrow

Smile and maybe tomorrow

you'll see the sun come shining through

for you.

Light up your face with gladness,

Hide every trace of sadness.

Although a tear may be ever so near

That's the time you must keep on trying.

Smile, what's the use of crying.

You'll see that life is still worthwhile – If you'll just

smile.

14 | Engaging Others Mindfully

… make me an instrument of your peace. Where there is hatred let me sow love.
St. Francis of Assisi

Getting chronic stress under control is both an internal and deliberate exercise. It requires taking time out to practice intentional breathing, to become familiar with the bodily sensations that inform you that stress has become chronic or that you're flooded, to reflect on your stories and mindset, and to treat your experience with humor and yourself with compassion and kindness. Even once you have these tools in hand, you aren't guaranteed that your relationships will flow smoothly. In fact, they may not. Engaging with others is work even under the best of circumstances.

Small and not so small disagreements, struggles, and conflict are inevitable. As you move through the world, you are bound to encounter others with viewpoints that differ from your own. You will be exposed to world events that sadden you, politicians that anger you, people who treat you poorly, and friends, family, and colleagues who push your buttons. Sometimes you may respond to them gracefully, and other times you may be flooded and reactive. What matters most is that you set an intention to engage each person mindfully, truthfully, and genuinely, and embody that commitment to the best of your ability.

People are typically attracted to those with whom they share common thoughts, feelings, values, and interests, and feel most connected to those with whom they agree. This means that we gauge the likability of others by how similar they are to us, and look to recreate ourselves in others as a way to confirm our stories and biases. In other words, we seek others who will prove that we are right. If we see ourselves as unworthy or unlovable, we are more likely to attract others who confirm that bias. If we embrace our goodness and value, we are more likely to be surrounded by those who bolster and support us.

One of the sources of dissatisfaction in relationship can be when others don't play by our rules. They may have different attitudes and beliefs. They may call into question our stories about ourselves and mindsets about how the world works. They also may not honor us or treat us with the kindness that we deserve. We may experience people who challenge our mindset as stressful, because interacting with them leads us to feel discomfort, frustration, irritation, anger, criticism, contempt, and avoidance. These reactions often harm or destroy our relationships. Part of our inability to accept dissimilarity in others is because we implicitly or explicitly expect that they *should* be similar. In response, we may assert or defend our viewpoint to prove that we are right. Being right is not necessarily in the best interest of the relationship. In fact, being right leaves little room for the other person to be in a relationship with us.

Fostering healthy relationships requires that we adopt a mindset of inclusion, accepting that others will come to us with their own stories and biases that are just as real for them as ours are for us. To coexist, we need to set an intention to soften the rigidity of our position and agree to be fully present and to listen and respond to others respectfully and without judgment. In her book, *The Bond*, journalist and author Lynne McTaggart states, "Engaging with another in any way obligates us to share the moment to the best of our ability, and to offer exactly what is required to help the other flourish…[This] changes the nature of the transaction between you and someone else from a selfish aim to a broader focus, whose whole purpose is the connection between the two of you…Once we view ourselves as part of a larger whole we begin to act differently toward each other. By removing a self-serving aim from the relationship, we stop fighting nature and surrender to our natural impulse toward holism. We can easily embrace difference within that larger definition of connection" (McTaggart 2012, p. 164).

Our primary goal in relationship is to take responsibility for our stress and emotional lives so that we can engage others mindfully, lovingly, and compassionately. As we learned in Part I, chronic stress severely undermines this capability. When flooded, it is difficult, if not impossible, to remain in the present moment and not default to unhelpful personal stories and habitual coping strategies. In a state of overwhelm, we are more likely to revert to primal defense strategies – attack/defend, avoid/flee, or ignore/freeze. Knowing this, we practice intentional breathing so that we can more readily relieve physiological stress, even in evocative situations.

Intentional breathing is just the first step. As you continue to explore the exercises in this book, you will become more aware of your stress level and when you are reaching the critical threshold of being flooded. You will also have a better sense of when you are operating at a high baseline level of stress by knowing where your body holds stress and intense emotion, and the physical cues that tell you that you're approaching a tipping point. Lastly, you will be more aware of the personal narratives and mindsets that you use to filter your experience, and be able to evaluate whether or not your stories are true or helpful for you in the present moment.

This may sound like a tall order at first, but with practice, these skills will become familiar to you on multiple levels – brain, body, and mind.

EXERCISE
Offering Kindness

A number of wisdom traditions use compassion or loving kindness practices to help cultivate feelings of gratitude, appreciation, respect, and love toward oneself and others. These practices typically begin with extending an intention of love towards oneself, then expanding the circle of compassion to include close others, strangers, and even those with whom we share contentious relationships. In using these practices in my own life and work, I have often found that it can seem easier to extend feelings of love to others. But, as you have learned during the course of this journey, you represent an amalgamation of neural networks, and highly complex matrices of thoughts, feelings, and bodily sensations, all of which were created to ensure your survival in some way. Learning to accept that your inherent nature is both remarkable yet flawed, allows you to move beyond expectations of perfection to embrace your physical and psychological asymmetries and imbalances, and to flow with life from that fundamental understanding.

Begin by making a commitment to take a purposeful pause for 10–20 minutes, during which you have no distraction. Then take approximately 3–5 minutes to relax your body and mind by practicing intentional breathing. Once you feel as though you have arrived in a place of relative calm, imagine yourself as a child or adult, then recite the following phrases slowly, and with intention.

May I be safe.

May I be happy.

May I be healthy.

May I be filled with ease.

Feel free to modify these words or create phrases that have meaning for you. As you repeat the words you choose, notice any thoughts, feelings, or sensations that arise in your mind and body. At times, you may feel at ease as you recite them, and at other times they may evoke feelings like sadness, anger, joy, or love. Whatever your experience, do your best to meet yourself with patience, kindness, and perhaps even a sense of humor, remembering that this is practice, and your task is to observe your response with as little judgment and as much compassion as possible.

After focusing on yourself for 5 or 10 minutes, begin to imagine someone in your life that you love or think of fondly. It may be a person from your past or present, alive or deceased. It may even be a cherished animal companion. Once you have decided on the person or being, bring their image to mind, and then slowly recite the following phrases:

May you be safe.

May you be happy.

May you be healthy.

May you be filled with ease.

Notice how it feels to recite these phrases to someone else. Is this experience similar to or different from your experience when you dedicated these phrases to yourself? If so, in what way? What did you learn from the experience?

The Great Ripple Effect

You may not think that your actions have consequences beyond the people that you know, love, or run into on the street, but experimenters in the fields of quantum physics, psi research, parapsychology, and other disciplines suggest otherwise. Their work indicates that your thoughts and actions may create a ripple effect, even at a distance. Talk about motivation for reducing stress and increasing your kindness quotient!

Psi researchers have long been interested in the effects of healing approaches such as telepathy, clairvoyance, psychokinesis, and precognition on health outcomes. In some studies, self-identified healers were asked to direct intentions for healing toward a particular animal or individual with a specified condition. Then changes in numerous biological systems in the recipient were measured while simultaneously ruling out self-regulation or the power of suggestion as potential counter explanations. A review and meta-analysis of 30 of these carefully controlled distance-healing studies supports the possibility that distance-healing intentions may affect their recipients (Schlitz & Braud 1997). The review's authors, Marilyn Schlitz and William Braud, leading experts in the field of alternative therapies, concluded that, in spite of a number of potential confounds and methodological considerations inherent in this line of research, "The statistical results are beyond what is expected by mean chance expectation. With relatively consistent findings from different laboratories, it is unlikely that the results are due to some systematic methodological flaws... In short, based on the standards applied to other areas of science, distant intentionality effects on biological systems, like other areas of psi research, appear promising for future inquiry" (Schlitz & Braud 1997, p. 71). We may never fully understand the nature or cause of these reported effects, however they raise the possibility that humans engage in forms of information exchange that go beyond our rational understanding.

In another example, authors of the "Love Study" sought to find out whether an average person, identified as a "sender," could affect the autonomic nervous system of a designated "receiver," simply through a directed intention (Radin et al. 2008). To do so, they recruited a sample of 36 dyads (72 participants), consisting of married couples, long-term partners, pairs of friends, and mothers and their child. In each case, one of the pair was being treated for cancer. Each dyad was randomly assigned to one of three groups: a trained distance-healing group (DHI), a waitlist DHI training group, and a no treatment control group.

Healthy partners in the DHI group and waitlist group were designated as the "sender" and the patient with cancer was designated as the "recipient." Senders in the DHI group attended an 8-hour, single-day group workshop that included instruction on the healing potential of compassionate intention, guided breath-based exercises to foster compassion (a Tibetan Buddhist practice called tonglen meditation), meditation and attention practices, Judeo-Christian meditation, and therapeutic touch. After the training session, DHI group members were asked to practice DHI mediation for three months, and to keep a daily log to document their practice. Following this practice period, pairs from all groups were invited to the laboratory to complete testing. Participants in the waitlist and no treatment control conditions were tested with no prior training.

Once in the laboratory, each member of a dyad was fixed with electrodes that measured physiological variables including skin conductance, heart rate, blood pressure, and respiration. Electrodermal activity (skin conductance) was the primary outcome of interest because it is considered a sensitive indicator of sympathetic nervous system activity, and relevant to the area of healing research. After each participant was fitted for physiological data collection, the pair was instructed to "maintain a feeling of connectedness with each other." They were then asked to exchange a personal item such as a watch or a ring and hold that object for the remainder of the session. The receiver was asked to sit in a reclining chair within a steel, double-walled, acoustically and electromagnetically shielded room and told that the sender would view random live video images of them sitting in the chair. The sender was then placed in a shielded room some 60 feet away and asked to "mentally connect" with the receiver as intensely as possible. Physiological instruments affixed to each person recorded any changes when the sender directed focused intention toward the receiver.

The electrodermal data revealed that a sender's intention had a measurable impact on the receiver's autonomic nervous system activity for all participants, regardless of whether or not they received training. While the overall effects were statistically small, the results suggested that intentions from senders in the DHI trained group had a slower, but more sustained effect on receivers, possibly because they had received prior training in focused attention, and compassion meditation. These effects were slightly smaller for the waitlist group, and smaller again for the control group. Although the study's authors were cautious in their interpretation of these results, they suggested that the healing intentions of one individual directed toward a close other may have direct physiological effects on the recipient (Radin et al. 2008). In other words, we may consciously or unconsciously experience the directed intentions of others, even at a distance (Radin et al. 2008), and this influence may be reciprocal (Radin 2006).

Although empirically rigorous research will be needed to convince the scientific community (including myself) of the veracity of energetic exchanges among people and groups, the potential implications of these ideas are staggering when we consider that we live in a culture characterized by high levels of stress, fear, aggression, and other intense emotions. There is considerable empirical support for the proposition that human behavior (Iacoboni 2009; Hatfield & Cacioppo 1994), social influence (Levy & Nail 1993), mood (Joiner & Katz 1999), emotional experience (Gump & Kulik 1997; Hatfield & Cacioppo 1994; Parkinson 2011), and stress (Gump & Kulik 1997), are contagious, and that this contagion may operate on a neural level (Iacoboni 2009; Christov-Moore & Iacoboni 2016). We have little understanding of how this process of contagion operates, however. What we do know is that our thoughts, feelings, and actions influence those around us and the social field in which we coexist, and that in the absence of managing our stress and other destructive emotions, we have the potential to inflict harm on those around us. This is one of the reasons why models like BREATHE are of such importance.

Being the Change

At some point in time you've likely observed contagion in the attitudes, emotions, and behaviors of the groups and organizations in which you participate. Sometimes it takes as little as one pessimistic individual to infuse an entire assembly of people with negativity. As we learned earlier, groups use stories and adopt mindsets to construct their reality, and these stories can have a ripple effect.

Groups experiencing high levels of stress operate similarly to individuals. Their process is marked by low self-awareness, emotional reactivity, inattention, fear-based decision-making, failure to accurately listen to or process information, cognitive rigidity, and an inability to recognize or challenge the stories that guide perception and action. This is part of the reason why countries wage war against each other. Governments enact oppressive policies. Men and women repress each other in the service of their perceived needs and interests. Companies mistreat workers. Banks engage in questionable practices to enhance their bottom line. And religious communities enforce their beliefs at the expense of individual freedom. When groups are stressed (and even when they are not) they can be blind to their own process, failing to question their mindsets, or examine the influence of stories on decision-making, policy, and action. That is, until someone has the courage to take a stand against them.

Insofar as there are those who cause harm, there are also those whose vocal opposition against the stories, mindsets, and behaviors of those in power change the course of human history. Mohandas Karamchand Gandhi, otherwise known as Mahatma Gandhi, was one such man. Gandhi is best known for his nonviolent stand against British colonizers in India, and his political activism aimed at attaining Indian self-governance, reducing poverty, decreasing ethnic and religious animosity, increasing women's rights, and attaining religious and political harmony. Often, his nonviolent protests left him in jail, where he continued to embody his intention to practice nonviolence. Gandhi was frequently accused of being overly passive and accommodating, refusing to endorse or support more aggressive means, yet he remained steadfast in his commitment to nonviolence. He was assassinated on January 30, 1948, and will always be known for his significant contribution to world peace as a nonviolent political and social activist.

Rosa Louise McCauley Parks, born in 1913 in Tuskegee, Alabama, was an African American civil rights activist, often referred to as the First Lady of the American Civil Rights Movement. On December 1, 1955, Parks refused to give up her bus seat in the "colored" section to a white passenger after the white section was filled. She was immediately arrested and charged with civil disobedience. Parks' nonviolent act of rebellion against a politically unjust system became an important catalyst for the American Civil Rights Movement. She spent the remainder of her life advocating for the rights of Black Americans and political prisoners, receiving numerous honors for her work including the Presidential Medal of Freedom and the Congressional Gold Medal. Her nonviolent defiance of racial discrimination went on to inspire future generations of leaders and activists.

Political activism is not reserved only for adults. Mattie Stepanek was a 13-year-old peace activist and author of the bestselling books, *Heartsongs* (2002) and *Just Peace:*

A Message of Hope (2008). Diagnosed with dysautonomic mitochondrial myopathy, a rare form of muscular dystrophy, Mattie realized that his time on this planet would be limited. Inspired by his hero, former U.S. President Jimmy Carter, Mattie made it his mission to promote peace, compassion, tolerance, and loving kindness. In spite of his physical suffering, he touched the lives of millions (including myself) through his luminous, wise, and unassuming presence. Mattie died in 2004 at the age of 13. His legacy is a mandate of hope and peace, and an example of someone committed to engaging others with loving kindness, even in the face of personal suffering.

Like Stepanek, Malala Yousafzai answered the call to stand up against hatred at an early age. She defied the oppressive dictates of the Taliban, who occupied her homeland of Pakistan, by demanding that girls be allowed to receive an education. In 2008, at age 11, she delivered a speech in Peshawar, Pakistan entitled, "How dare the Taliban take away my basic right to education?" She then became a blogger for the British Broadcasting Corporation (BBC), raising the world's consciousness about the plight of young women being attacked in their schools by Taliban rebels. In 2012, an armed terrorist boarded her school bus and shot her in the head, nearly ending her life. She addressed the United Nations on her sixteenth birthday in 2013, and authored an autobiography entitled, *I Am Malala: The Girl Who Stood Up For Education and Was Shot By The Taliban* (2015). In spite of continued Taliban threats, Malala remains a staunch and vocal advocate for educational rights. She was awarded the Nobel Peace Prize in 2014, becoming the youngest person to ever receive that honor.

There are many men, women, and children who use their gifts of speech, action, and artistry to advocate for a peaceful, diplomatic, non-military, and philosophical resolution to the world's problems. These individuals set an example for what is possible when we take responsibility for ourselves and the systems that impact our lives, question the stories that are being told, and, as needed, take action against them.

Being the Change in Your Life

You may be asking yourself, "What do the lives of activists have to do with my life and its stressors?" First off, helping others can reduce your stress level. Studies show that acts of giving stimulate the same neural regions in the brain that regulate the stress response. These regions have inhibitory connections with areas of the brain's limbic system and related structures known to be involved in reacting to stress and threat. Giving social support is associated with decreased stress-related activity in the dorsal anterior cingulate cortex, anterior insula, and amygdala, all regions that are highly activated when processing stressful stimuli. Offering support to others is also linked to reduced vulnerability to negative psychological outcomes (Inagaki et al. 2016). This dampening of the stress response following giving behavior may explain studies that link altruism with better health and lower mortality rates (Post 2007). In essence, giving to others may help reduce your stress and enhance your health and wellbeing.

Second, as we saw in the first chapter, social connection is good for you. You may interact with others through writing, educating, designing technology that improves lives, healing, cooking, cleaning, caring for the earth, nurturing or supporting family members or friends, or using any number of talents that you uniquely possess. Or you may set an intention to greet others kindly and respectfully, and offer a helping hand whenever the opportunity arises. Whatever you choose, small acts of grace go a long way in reducing your stress and improving your life and those of others.

Over 25 years ago, I picked up a wonderful little book that changed the way that I view others. The book, *A Policy of Kindness*, introduced some of the teachings of His Holiness the Dalai Lama about peace, compassion, and nonviolence (Piburn 1990). It offered a perspective about the human condition, and the fact that each of us has similar wishes and desires, regardless of where we come from. The Dalai Lama says, "The realization that we are all basically the same human beings, who seek happiness and try to avoid suffering, is very helpful in developing a sense of brotherhood and sisterhood – a warm feeling of love and compassion for others. This, in turn, is essential if we are to survive in this ever-shrinking world we live in. For if we each selfishly pursue only what we believe to be in our own interest, without caring for the needs of others, we not only may end up harming others but also ourselves" (Piburn 1990, p. 16).

Your story need not be as public as those of Mahatma Gandhi or Malala Yousafzai, but its impact on your wellbeing, and those with whom you live and work, is no less important. When you greet another being with respect and kindness, you feed that energy forward. People who are treated with appreciation and thoughtfulness tend to treat others similarly. Just as negativity is contagious, so is kindness. Each time you interact with other people or beings, ask yourself, "How can I be the change that I want to see in the world?" If you take the time to pause, reduce your level of stress, turn down the volume of your mental chatter, and listen to the innermost longings of your heart and mind, you may be amazed what you discover.

15 | BREATHE in Action

The best way out is always through.

Robert Frost

The BREATHE model is predicated on five key assumptions. First, mindfulness is inherently relational. From neurons to vast global networks, you build mindfulness through the matrices of meaning that you create, and the relationships and systems you form that embody that meaning.

Second, chronic stress undermines your health, happiness, and capacity to live mindfully. When chronically stressed, your sympathetic nervous system (SNS) is dominant, increasing emotional and behavioral reactivity, and amplifying the probability that you will rely on your habitual stories as lenses of perception. This may lead to distorted appraisals, particularly when your stories are negative. Moreover, chronic stress leads to reduced self-regulation and suppressed cognitive resources and coping skills. In combination, these factors can impair your capacity to function and communicate effectively, and may erode the foundation of your relationships.

Third, the breath is the gateway to mindfulness. When in a state of physiological homeostasis you are more able to be aware of and attend to the present, and adopt a mindset of acceptance and nonjudgment. This, in turn, allows you to listen and communicate effectively, and to build satisfying social bonds. Intentional breathing is an effective tool for balancing the autonomic nervous system (ANS) and attaining this equilibrium.

Fourth, the stories you tell shape your life. In examining your narratives you can recognize how you construe and construct your experience, and appraise, accept, challenge, or refute these stories, rather than be governed by them. Then you become able to respond to your circumstances based on present events, rather than reacting from past wounds or future expectations.

Finally, mindfulness is a practice. It requires time and space to care for yourself and to become familiar with the workings of your mind and body. The more you are able to loosen the reins of perfectionism, accept your humanity in its many forms, and to laugh at your foibles, face plants, and idiosyncrasies, the less suffering you will create. From here you can practice engaging yourself and others mindfully, and with acceptance and compassion (Figure 15.1).

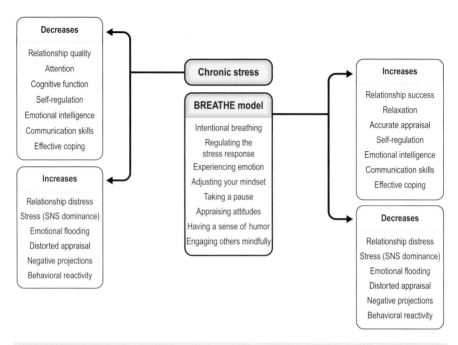

Figure 15.1

Summary of BREATHE Model

The Seven Skills of BREATHE are tools that will allow you to achieve these goals. They include:

1. **B**REATH AWARENESS: Becoming aware of your mechanics of breathing. This is the first step in the process of learning how to use your breath. Eventually, breathing deeply and fully becomes habitual rather than volitional. Similar to learning how to ride a bike, it takes time and repetition for your brain and body to coordinate this new way of breathing.

2. **R**EGULATING your autonomic nervous system through the practice of intentional breathing. Practice intentional breathing as frequently as possible (at least several times per day). As intentional breathing becomes more familiar, you will observe your breath pattern changing and find it easier to recruit your breath for relaxation whenever you choose – even during stressful encounters with others.

3. **E**XPERIENCING emotions, rather than suppressing them. As you become familiar with your emotional landscape, you will be empowered to choose how to express or regulate your feelings.

4. **A**PPRAISING your mindset and the stories that you tell about yourself is key to managing your thoughts, feelings, and behaviors. Exploring these stories will yield tremendous insight into the assumptions that drive how you relate to yourself and others. The more cognizant you are of these stories, the more able you will be to challenge their assumptions and rewrite new stories that reflect the present moment, rather than the past or future.

5. **T**AKING purposeful pauses. Making time for yourself will allow you to explore intentional breathing, to reduce your level of stress, to experience your emotional world fully, to examine your stories, attitudes, and mindsets, and to allow yourself to rest and repair. This can seem like the most challenging task, particularly at first, yet it is essential to create sustainable change in your life and relationships.

6. **H**UMOR is a necessary ingredient in all of life's adventures. Although relationships often feel like serious business, the extent to which you can treat yourself with loving kindness, cut yourself some slack, embrace your imperfections, and do the same for others, will make a huge difference in the quality of your experience.

7. **E**NGAGING others differently. It is one thing to sit in a room, breathe intentionally, become self-aware, and feel attuned to your experience. Engaging others differently requires making a commitment to practicing these skills when you are emotionally aroused, physiologically flooded, or feeling overwhelmed by life stress. That is the true measure of being present in relationship, and it is part of a continuous and evolutionary process in which we are willing to both succeed and fall on our faces over and over again. It is the process of being alive in all of its grief and glory.

Taking Action – Creating a Legacy Statement

Setting an intention to meet the world mindfully is no easy task. As you practice the skills in the BREATHE model, you will become familiar with your stress cues, emotional responses, and the stories that shape your experience. Once you begin to pause, evaluate your circumstances, and put the BREATHE practices to work, you may notice that a whole new set of questions emerge. Many of my clients, students, and workshop participants report a tendency to re-evaluate their lives while engaging in this process. Questions like, "Who am I?" "What do I want?" "Why am I here?" and, "What really matters?" often surface. It is natural that questions will arise as you explore reducing stress, get to know your mind and body better, and observe and potentially rewrite your personal story.

Some of the best advice I have heard on setting intentions comes from Steven Covey, author of *The Seven Habits of Highly Effective People* (1989). Covey writes, "Begin with the end in mind." I have found that one of the most powerful strategies for uncovering your sense of purpose, and altering your course, is to consider what you would like your legacy to be when you leave this earth. Once you know what legacy you would like to leave, you can work backwards to create a plan of action to fulfill your vision.

> **EXERCISE**
> **My Legacy Statement**
>
> In Chapter 11, you completed an exercise in which you identified the core values that shape your life. Turn back to that exercise and write down the top five values that you identified. Don't worry if you end up with more or fewer, or if your priorities have shifted since then. See if you can come up with five to seven at the most. Take a few moments to review those values and their importance in your life. Then find a comfortable place where you

can sit undisturbed for at least 15–20 minutes. Slowly begin to draw your awareness to your breath, just as it is. From that place, begin your practice of intentional breathing, inhaling deeply and fully, and exhaling slowly.

Once you feel settled in the present moment, imagine that you have one more day to live. Envision the experience in as much detail as you like, perhaps imagining who you would choose to be with, and where you would feel most happy and comfortable. Once you are settled in that image, begin to write down your responses to the following questions.

How would you describe yourself?

What are your greatest accomplishments?

What are your biggest regrets?

What would you most like others to remember about you?

Take a few moments to write down your responses to these questions as mindfully as you are able to in this moment. You can always come back and add more later.

Once you finish this exercise, read over what you have written. Then take some time to reflect on the following questions.

What am I doing right now that is allowing me to manifest my desired legacy?

What I am doing that does not contribute to my desired legacy?

Is there anything that I might do differently?

How may I be the change that I want to see in my own life?

How may I be the change that I want to see in the lives of others?

This statement is a work in progress. You may discover that you are well on your way to creating the legacy that you envision. You may also notice that there are discrepancies between your envisioned legacy and the path that you are on now. That is good information. Consider it a form of eustress – a perturbation that prompts you to consider changing your habits, stories, mindset, or way of being, to reflect your deepest values and priorities. The good news is you can do something about it. You can begin by setting an intention to do something differently. Life is a practice. Each day, you can move in the direction of being the person you envision yourself to be, continue to be the amazing person you are, or both.

Creating an Intention That Leads to Action

Whatever legacy you choose, the first step involves setting an intention to take responsibility for yourself and your life, and creating an action plan that leads you toward success. From that foundation, you are more able to engage relationships mindfully.

An action plan is a contract that you make with yourself. It is a commitment to incorporate practices such as the seven skills of BREATHE into your life on a continuous basis. The seven skills are an excellent foundation to support you on your journey.

> **EXERCISE**
> **Creating an Action Plan**
>
> Create an action plan for yourself that reflects three to five steps that you are willing to take in the next month. Then commit to doing at least one thing on this list every day for the next 30 days. Your action steps may include:
>
> 1. Practicing intentional breathing for three to five minutes at least twice a day.
> 2. Taking a purposeful pause to do something that nurtures me (e.g. taking a walk or a yoga class, reading a book, speaking with a supportive friend, doing something fun, and examining what I really want from my life).
> 3. Writing my personal stories in a journal.
> 4. Spending 15 minutes each day listening to a significant person without any outside or technological distractions.
> 5. Sitting in stillness and becoming familiar with myself.
>
> Write down your action steps as a contract, then sign and date the document. Place the list in a prominent position in your home, like on your refrigerator or bathroom mirror. Each time you complete an action, place a check mark next to it to monitor your progress.

Just Like Me

I end each of my teachings and workshops with this exercise. It is designed to remind us of the similarities that we all share as we navigate our world, and to kindle a bit more compassion and loving kindness in our hearts.

> **EXERCISE**
> **Just Like Me**
>
> You can do this exercise with a partner in a dyad, or on your own by imagining that there is someone in front of you. Become aware of that person – a fellow human being, just like you. Now silently repeat these phrases, while looking at or imagining your partner.
>
> This person has a body and a mind, just like me.
>
> This person has feelings, emotions, and thoughts, just like me.
>
> This person has experienced physical and emotional pain and suffering, just like me.

This person has at some point been sad, disappointed, angry, or hurt, just like me.

This person has felt unworthy or inadequate, just like me.

This person worries and is frightened sometimes, just like me.

This person has longed for friendship, just like me.

This person is learning about life, just like me.

This person wants to be caring and kind to others, just like me.

This person wants to be content with what life has given, just like me.

This person wishes to be free from pain and suffering, just like me.

This person wishes to be safe and healthy, just like me.

This person wishes to be happy, just like me.

This person wishes to be loved, just like me.

Now, allow some wishes for wellbeing to arise:

I wish that this person has the strength, resources, and social support to navigate the difficulties in life with ease.

I wish that this person be free from pain and suffering.

I wish that this person be peaceful and happy.

I wish that this person be loved.

Because this person is a fellow human being, just like me.

After a few moments, thank your partner with a bow or in whatever way feels appropriate.

There are many ways to practice the Just Like Me exercise. When on your own, conjure up the image of a person you love, like, or even dislike and repeat these phrases to yourself. When standing in line, on a bus or subway or in a public place, try repeating these phrases. You don't need to remember them perfectly. Any approximation will do.

This is also a very powerful exercise to do in families, groups, organizations and other contexts in which people gather. Choose a partner and repeat these words in your mind to each other. In realizing our common needs and longings, we can begin to create a world of "us-ing" instead of othering. We can choose peace over conflict and mindfulness over stress-driven reactivity. You have the power to shape your destiny. What will you create?

A courageous heart will go forth and engage with life despite confusion and fear.

A fearful heart will be hesitant and will tend to hold back.

A heavy heart will make for a gloomy, unlived life.

A compassionate heart need never carry the burden of judgment.

A forgiving heart knows the art of liberation.

A loving heart awakens the spirit of possibility and engagement with others.

By John O'Donohue

Exercises

EXERCISE
How Stressed Do You Feel?

The following is a survey, The Perceived Stress Scale, which assesses your current level of stress. Take a few moments to complete the questions. What did you learn?

The questions in this scale ask you about your feelings and thoughts during the last month. In each case, please choose the number from 0–4 that reflects how often you felt or thought a certain way.

0 = Never 1 = Almost Never 2 = Sometimes 3 = Fairly Often 4 = Very Often

1. In the last month, how often have you been upset because of something that happened unexpectedly?

2. In the last month, how often have you felt that you were unable to control the important things in your life?

3. In the last month, how often have you felt nervous and "stressed"?

4. In the last month, how often have you felt confident about your ability to handle your personal problems?

5. In the last month, how often have you felt that things were going your way?

6. In the last month, how often have you found that you could not cope with all the things that you had to do?

7. In the last month, how often have you been able to control irritations in your life?

8. In the last month, how often have you felt that you were on top of things?

9. In the last month, how often have you been angered because of things that were outside of your control?

10. In the last month, how often have you felt difficulties were piling up so high that you could not overcome them?

Cohen S, Kamarck T, Mermelstein R (1983) A global measure of perceived stress. Journal of Health and Social Behavior 24:386–396

EXERCISE
Identifying Your Personal Story

Take a few moments to write down your personal (or organizational) story. You may use simple descriptive phrases like, "I am tough," "I take care of others before myself," "I am good at math."

You may also choose to write down experiences, family beliefs or other influences that helped to shape how you view yourself now. Once you have listed your beliefs about yourself, and identified a few of your stories, look at each one and ask yourself the following questions:

1. Where did this story come from?

2. Is this my story or someone else's?

3. Is this story true of me now?

4. Is this story contributing to or undermining my happiness?

5. Do I choose to continue to live this story or is it time to write a new one?

EXERCISE
Becoming Aware of Your Breath

The following practice introduces a simple yet effective technique to become attuned to your breath. The emphasis here is on observing how you breathe and beginning to become familiar with the breath's sensation. Remember that this is a practice. It may feel strange, awkward, or difficult, and you may or may not be able to sense a great deal at first. Don't worry. These feelings are common when you aren't used to sensing what is going on in your physical body. Be kind to yourself and remember that this is an exploration. Also remember that if, for any reason, you feel really uncomfortable or this doesn't feel right to you, take a break, and try again another time.

First, find a quiet place where you can sit for roughly 10 minutes without interruption. If you're worried about turning off your phone or shutting your spouse, children, dogs, cats, or other companions out of the room, don't be. They will be just fine without you for 10 minutes. Trust me, I've been there.

Now assume a comfortable position like sitting upright in a chair or lying on your back. If you're sleepy, I'd suggest sitting up or this may turn into a nap.

Begin to observe your breath just as it is. Notice where you are breathing into – upper chest, front, back, or sides. There are no right or wrong ways to breathe – just observe for a few minutes. Once you get familiar with the flow of your breath, you may want to consider a few of these questions.

How does your breath feel as you breathe in and out? It is shallow or deep?

Is it easy to breathe or does it take effort?

Does your breath flow smoothly in and out or does it feel as though it gets stuck in some places?

Does it tend to move into the front or back or sides of your torso?

What is the pace of your breath? Does it seem typical or is it faster or slower than what you usually experience?

Has your breathing changed since you started observing it?

Do you notice any other sensations in addition to your breath?

Continue to observe the sensations for a few more minutes, noticing any feelings or thoughts that arise. Most importantly, try to become familiar with the rhythm and flow of your breath while remaining comfortable and relaxed. This may be the first time that you've paid much attention to the subtleties of your breathing. If it feels strange or you feel a bit anxious or uncomfortable, rest assured that your feelings are typical. Most new experiences make us uneasy.

Once you've spent 3–5 minutes becoming familiar with your breathing, pause and take a break. Then reflect on some of the questions above and your experience. Did you learn anything new about your breathing or about yourself?

EXERCISE
Intentional Breathing

The following practice introduces a simple yet effective form of deep breathing called intentional breathing. Unlike other techniques of "belly" or "abdominal" breathing, the emphasis here is to allow the natural flow of the breath by inhaling from the top down and exhaling from the bottom up. Before you begin, a couple of things to remember:

First, this is a practice. It may feel strange, awkward, or difficult. That is to be expected when trying something that you've never attempted before. Be kind with yourself and see this as an exploration rather than something to be immediately mastered. Second, and more importantly, if for any reason you feel really uncomfortable or this doesn't feel right to you, it is perfectly OK to take a break or discontinue the exercise and try again another time.

Begin by finding a comfortable position like sitting upright in a chair or lying on your back. Begin to observe your breath just as it is. Notice where the breath flows – upper chest, lower belly, front, back, or sides. As you do, try to avoid placing a judgment on how you are breathing or attaching a story to it. Just as if you were a scientist studying a cell under a microscope, see if you can examine all of the details of your breath one at a time and make mental notes of them.

Observe how you are breathing just as you are. It's an interesting exercise. You may already notice that the act of observing your breath slows down your respiration rate.

Next, place your right hand on your breastbone (sternum) in the center of your chest.

Place your left hand so that your thumb is below your navel. Continue to breathe normally and observe whether you are breathing more into your right hand or left hand. See if you can resist the urge to change your breath or make it deeper. Breathe as normally as you can and observe how it is to be in your body, breathing normally. How does it feel? What do you notice? Continue for at least 10 breaths.

Now try breathing just into your right hand that is resting in the middle of your upper chest. Without forcing the breath, see how it feels to breathe into the space below your right hand. What do you notice? Can you slow your inhalation or is that difficult or uncomfortable? Just see what happens. Keep observing for 10–20 breaths. After 10–20 breaths, take a few deep inhalations and exhalations and resume breathing normally for a minute or so.

Next try breathing just into your left hand that is resting on your lower abdomen. Without forcing the breath, see how it feels to breathe into the space below your left hand. What do you notice? Can you slow your inhalation or is that difficult or uncomfortable? Just see what happens. Keep observing for 10–20 breaths. After 10–20 breaths, take a few deep inhalations and exhalations and resume breathing normally for a minute or so.

Now try breathing half of your inhalation into your right hand, pause for a second or two, and then breathe the remainder into the space below your left hand and pause. Then exhale from the bottom up, first releasing the air below your left hand, then allowing the exhalation to continue from below your left hand to below your right hand, traveling up and out either through your nose or mouth. Continue to your next inhalation, first into the area beneath your right hand and then into the area beneath your left hand, then exhale from the bottom up. Can you slow your inhalation or is that difficult or uncomfortable? How does it feel? What do you notice? Keep observing for 10–20 breaths. After 10–20 breaths, take a few deep inhalations and exhalations and resume breathing normally for a minute or so.

Finally, try breathing deeply and fully from top to bottom as you inhale and bottom to top as you exhale without pausing. If possible, see if you can slow the exhalation so that it is longer than the inhalation. If you like, you can count 1, 2, 3, and so on to see which is longer, your inhalation or your exhalation. After 10–20 breaths, take a few big deep inhalations and exhalations and resume breathing normally for a minute or so.

Notice how you feel. Was the exercise simple or difficult? Did breathing slowly and fully seem usual to you? How do you feel physically? Emotionally? Energetically? If you like, write down your experience.

This exercise is intended to activate your parasympathetic nervous system and elicit the relaxation response. While not everyone experiences relaxation right away, most report feeling a sense of calm and a reduction in the feeling of stress following this exercise. Now, for fun, take in a deep breath and try singing "om" using a single tone again and count how long you hold the tone. Do you see a difference? Most people do!

For an audio recording of the Intentional Breathing Exercise see www.bgracebullock.com.

EXERCISE
Experiencing Your Heart

Place one or both of your hands over your heart (on your chest to the left of your breastbone). Close your eyes or cast your gaze downward away from distraction.

Take a few moments to see if you can feel your heartbeat. This may be easy or difficult depending on your familiarity with your body. Once you find it, observe the beating of your heart just as it is. What do you notice?

Does your heartbeat seem fast or slow?

Is it pounding or beating calmly?

Is your heartbeat regular or irregular?

Does it speed up, slow down, or maintain a consistent pace?

Is there anything else that you notice about it?

Take a few moments to write down your experience.

EXERCISE
Attuning to Your Body

The following exercise uses intentional breathing to attune to where you may hold emotions in your body. Remember that this is a practice. It may feel strange, awkward, or difficult, and you may or may not be able to experience your emotions as bodily sensations. This is not unusual. We are often disconnected from the experience of our physical bodies, so it can take time and practice to develop that awareness. Remember that this is an exploration. If for any reason you feel uncomfortable or need to discontinue this exercise, take a break, and come back to it at another time.

First, find a quiet place where you can sit for roughly 10 minutes without interruption. Find a comfortable position sitting upright in a chair or lying on your back. If you're sleepy, I recommend sitting. Once you are comfortable, begin to breathe intentionally as you've practiced previously. Breathe into the heart area first and then down into the lower abdomen as fully and deeply as you are able, then exhale slowly, as if you are deflating the air out of a balloon from the bottom up. Once you find a comfortable rhythm, observe your breath for another few minutes as you move into a deeper state of relaxation.

Once you are breathing comfortably, shift your attention to your body. How does your body feel overall? What do you notice? Are there places where you feel tension or restriction? Are there areas of your body that are more relaxed? Are there any sensations that you feel more strongly? Focus your attention on whatever sensation you feel most strongly in your body right now. It may be very subtle or quite noticeable. Where is the sensation located? Once you've identified a location, give it your full attention for a few minutes.

Then shift your focus to the quality of that sensation. Can you find words to describe it like sharp, dull, tight, loose, stiff, throbbing, hot, cold, uncomfortable, or painful? Does this sensation remain in one place? Does it shift or change? See if you can keep your mind on the sensation and resist the urge to create stories around it. Notice how it feels and allow that feeling to be present without trying to alter it or describe it beyond a few words. What happens when you stay focused on that sensation for a while? Is there anything else that you notice about it? Do other sensations arise as well?

Then notice whether you feel any particular emotions while focusing on that sensation. As we learned above, our bodies store a great deal of information, often providing messages and clues about how we are feeling. What emotion or emotions, if any, do you feel when focusing in on that sensation? Remember, there are no right or wrong answers. You may feel strong emotions like anger, sadness, grief, joy, or serenity, or you may feel very little. It can take practice to become familiar with our body sensations and the emotions that they evoke. This is just a first step.

Continue to observe the sensation and the emotions that you experience for a few more minutes. Do the feelings stay the same? Do they shift or change to other emotions? Are they pleasant or unpleasant? Do you feel comfortable paying attention to the feelings or experience the desire to shift your focus? Once you've spent about 5 minutes getting familiar with these sensations and any feelings that arise, take a break. Then reflect on the questions above and your experience while doing this exercise. Did you learn anything new about yourself?

EXERCISE
Exploring Your Appraisal and Coping Style

Find a quiet place where you can sit for roughly 10–15 minutes without interruption. Take a few moments to practice the intentional breathing exercise in Chapter 9. Once you feel comfortable and relaxed, bring your attention to one challenging or demanding circumstance in your life – your bills, kids, job, parents, or spouse. Imagine that person or situation in as much detail as you can, including your thoughts, feelings, stories about the situation, and any sensations that you feel in your body. Then ask yourself the following questions. Take a few minutes to write down your responses:

What comes to mind when I think of this person or situation?

Do I feel physically or emotionally tense or uncomfortable?

Where do I experience sensations in my body?

Do I excessively ruminate or worry about this situation or person?

What is my story about this person or circumstance?

How does that story relate to any of my other personal stories?

How do I cope with this challenge?

Do I avoid the person or circumstance altogether or wish it would just go away?

Do I confront the problem head on and do my best to change things?

Do I feel able to change the situation or do I feel powerless or incompetent?

How do my feelings of being empowered or powerless relate to whether or not I experience this circumstance or person as stressful?

What did I learn from this exercise?

EXERCISE
Working with Your Stories

Most of the time, when confronted with interpersonal conflict or other stressors, we avoid, resist, confront, or catastrophize. This reaction is habitual. You may not even be aware of it at first. It's not that this response is bad. It is a coping mechanism that you developed early in life, and with repeated practice it became second nature. However, in the present, it may be unskillful or potentially destructive to your personal and professional relationships. Although it can be extremely uncomfortable, your discomfort zone creates the opportunity to re-appraise your circumstances and ask yourself, "Does the situation trigger a negative or unhelpful personal story?"

Sometimes identifying a story is easier than you think. Take a moment to recall a very recent stressful experience that you shared with another person. Try to remember the event as vividly as you can.

Now write down your response to the following questions.

What personal story or belief did I tell myself during this experience? (e.g. "I am a good person," "I am a failure," "I make everyone happy at my own expense," "I should be nice no matter what," "Nobody likes me," "I need to be right.")

Is that story true for me now?

Do I want to continue living this story?

Questioning your story can and often does initiate a process of re-appraisal. Re-appraisal involves questioning your attitudes, attributions, and your story's role in shaping them. From here, you may view situations differently and find alternative responses.

EXERCISE
Reappraising Your Story

Take some time to write down three situations or people in your life that you are struggling with or that you experience as stressful. It can be a situation or person at work or involve family or friends, your neighbors, or even your dog or cat. Just think of three things that are driving you nuts and write them down. Don't censor yourself. There is no right or wrong answer. Just write.

Once you've identified three situations, pick one and write down your responses to the following questions.

1. How much does this situation/person bother me?

1= not at all; 2= a little bit; 3= somewhat; 4 = quite a bit; 5= very much

2. What personal story am I telling myself around this situation/person?

3. What is my typical response to the situation/person?

4. Do I have the ability to change the circumstances?

5. Can I think about this situation/person differently?

6. Can I react to this situation/person differently? If so, how?

7. Am I willing to change my thoughts about the situation?

8. Am I willing to change my feelings about the situation?

9. Am I willing to respond to the situation differently?

10. How much of this situation is about me? How much is about the other person?

11. How much of this is my responsibility to change?

Now look back at your responses and see whether you can detect any themes in your stories. What do these themes or stories tell you about yourself? If you'd like, try the exercise again for the other two situations that you identified.

EXERCISE
Exploring Your Values

Begin with a few minutes of intentional breathing to bring yourself into the present moment.

Now take a look at the list below and circle your top ten values. This list is not exhaustive.

If something is missing, please feel free to add it.

Once you've identified your top 10, spend a few moments identifying your top three most preferred values.

List of Values

Acceptance	Creativity	Hard work
Accountability	Curiosity	Harmony
Achievement	Dialogue	Health
Adaptability	Discipline	Helping others
Ambition	Discovery	Honesty
Artistry	Ease with uncertainty	Humility
Attitude	Enthusiasm	Humor/fun
Awareness	Entrepreneurial	Inclusion
Balance (home/work)	Environmental sustainability	Independence
Beauty	Equality	Ingenuity
Being the best	Ethics	Integrity
Caring	Excellence	Interdependence
Coaching / mentoring	Fairness	Initiative
Commitment	Family	Innovation
Community involvement	Financial stability	Intuition
Compassion	Forgiveness	Job security
Competence	Friendships	Leadership
Conflict resolution	Freedom	Learning
Continuous learning	Fun	Listening
Cooperation	Future generations	Making a difference
Courage	Generosity	Mental sharpness
Creating peace	Gratitude	Mindfulness
	Happiness	Nature

Open communication	Recognition	Strength
Openness	Reliability	Success
Patience	Resourcefulness	Teamwork
Perseverance	Respect	Trust
Personal fulfillment	Responsibility	Vision
Personal growth	Risk-taking	Wealth
Physical achievement	Safety	Wellbeing
Physical strength	Self-discipline	Willpower
Power	Social justice	Wisdom
Professional growth	Spiritual growth	World peace

Once you have identified your top three, pick one and write your responses to the following questions. As you explore these answers remember that the purpose of the exercise isn't to evaluate how "good" you are at living up to these values and aspirations.

This exercise is intended to get you in touch with your deepest values and how they may or may not influence your current story, decisions, and actions.

1. Why is this value most important to you?

2. How does this value affect how you treat yourself?

3. How does this value affect how you treat others?

4. How does this value guide your decision-making?

5. Is this value reflected in your personal story? How?

6. Is this your value or one that was given to you by someone else?

EXERCISE
Rewriting Your Story

Take some time in a quiet place to reflect on the story that you would like to write for yourself. It could be a story of who you are, who you would like to become, who you would like to be in relationships with family, close friends, your spouse or partner, or your colleagues. If you find that it seems like a big undertaking to rewrite or revise your story, consider looking at your responses to the values exercise above and see if you can rewrite your story in a way that reflects your top values.

EXERCISE
Holding the Space

Find a place where you will not be distracted or interrupted for about 5–10 minutes. Leave your mobile devices behind (preferably turn them off). Once you are seated comfortably, sit upright, lengthen your spine while keeping your face, neck, and shoulders relaxed. Then close your eyes or turn your gaze downward to reduce distraction. Then sit silently and still for 3–5 minutes.

Once you are done, explore the following questions.

How did it feel to sit and do nothing?

How did it feel to be in silence?

What physical sensations did you notice?

Did your experience of sensations, thoughts, or feelings change as time passed?

Did you feel the need to do something, think about something, run a story through your mind, create a list, problem-solve, plan an activity, or something else?

Did sitting and doing nothing in silence with no particular agenda feel comfortable or uncomfortable?

Remember that there are no right or wrong answers. You are gathering information about your experience.

A number of wisdom traditions use compassion or loving kindness practices to help cultivate feelings of gratitude, appreciation, respect, and love toward oneself and others. These practices typically begin with extending an intention of love towards oneself, then expanding the circle of compassion to include close others, strangers, and even those with whom we share contentious relationships. In using these practices in my own life and work, I have often found that it can seem easier to extend feelings of love to others. But, as you have learned during the course of this journey, you represent an amalgamation of neural networks, and highly complex matrices of thoughts, feelings, and bodily sensations, all of which were created to ensure your survival in some way. Learning to accept that your inherent nature is both remarkable yet flawed, allows you to move beyond expectations of perfection to embrace your physical and psychological asymmetries and imbalances, and to flow with life from that fundamental understanding.

Begin by making a commitment to take a purposeful pause for 10–20 minutes, during which you have no distraction. Then take approximately 3–5 minutes to relax your body and mind by practicing intentional breathing. Once you feel as though you have arrived in a place of relative calm, imagine yourself as a child or adult, then recite the following phrases slowly, and with intention.

May I be safe.

May I be happy.

May I be healthy.

May I be filled with ease.

Feel free to modify these words, or create phrases that have meaning for you. As you repeat the words you choose, notice any thoughts, feelings, or sensations that arise in your mind and body. At times, you may feel at ease as you recite them, and at other times they may evoke feelings like sadness, anger, joy, or love. Whatever your experience, do your best to meet yourself with patience, kindness, and perhaps even a sense of humor, remembering that this is practice, and your task is to observe your response with as little judgment and as much compassion as possible.

After focusing on yourself for 5–10 minutes, begin to imagine someone in your life that you love or think of fondly. It may be a person from your past or present, alive or deceased. It may even be a cherished animal companion. Once you have decided on the person or being, bring their image to mind, and then slowly recite the following phrases:

May you be safe.

May you be happy.

May you be healthy.

May you be filled with ease.

Notice how it feels to recite these phrases to someone else. Is this experience similar to or different from your experience when you dedicated these phrases to yourself? If so, in what way? What did you learn from the experience?

EXERCISE
My Legacy Statement

In Chapter 11, you completed an exercise in which you identified the core values that shape your life. Turn back to that exercise and write down the top five values that you identified. Don't worry if you end up with more or fewer, or if your priorities have shifted since then. See if you can come up with five to seven at the most. Take a few moments to review those values and their importance in your life. Then find a comfortable place where you can sit undisturbed for at least 15–20 minutes. Slowly begin to draw your awareness to your breath, just as it is. From that place, begin your practice of intentional breathing, inhaling deeply and fully and exhaling slowly.

Once you feel settled in the present moment, imagine that you have one more day to live. Envision the experience in as much detail as you like, perhaps imagining who you would choose to be with, and where you would feel most happy and comfortable. Once you are settled in that image, begin to write down your responses to the following questions.

How would you describe yourself?

What are your greatest accomplishments?

What are your biggest regrets?

What would you most like others to remember about you?

Take a few moments to write down your responses to these questions as mindfully as you are able to in this moment. You can always come back and add more later.

Once you finish this exercise, read over what you have written. Then take some time to reflect on the following questions.

What am I doing right now that is allowing me to manifest my desired legacy?

What I am doing that does not contribute to my desired legacy?

Is there anything that I might do differently?

How may I be the change that I want to see in my own life?

How may I be the change that I want to see in the lives of others?

EXERCISE
Creating an Action Plan

Create an action plan for yourself that reflects three to five steps that you are willing to take in the next month. Then commit to doing at least one thing on this list every day for the next 30 days. Your action steps may include.

1. Practicing intentional breathing for 3–5 minutes at least twice a day.

2. Taking a purposeful pause to do something that nurtures me (e.g. taking a walk or a yoga class, reading a book, speaking with a supportive friend, doing something fun, examining what I really want from my life…).

3. Writing my personal stories in a journal.

4. Spending 15 minutes each day listening to a significant person without any outside or technological distractions.

5. Sitting in stillness and becoming familiar with myself.

Write down your action steps as a contract, then sign and date the document. Place the list in a prominent position in your home, like on your refrigerator or bathroom mirror. Each time you complete an action, place a check mark next to it to monitor your progress.

EXERCISE
Just Like Me

You can do this exercise with a partner in a dyad, or on your own by imagining that there is someone in front of you. Become aware of that person – a fellow human being, just like you. Now silently repeat these phrases, while looking at, or imagining your partner.

This person has a body and a mind, just like me.

This person has feelings, emotions, and thoughts, just like me.

This person has experienced physical and emotional pain and suffering, just like me.

This person has at some point been sad, disappointed, angry, or hurt, just like me.

This person has felt unworthy or inadequate, just like me.

This person worries and is frightened sometimes, just like me.

This person has longed for friendship, just like me.

This person is learning about life, just like me.

This person wants to be caring and kind to others, just like me.

This person wants to be content with what life has given, just like me.

This person wishes to be free from pain and suffering, just like me.

This person wishes to be safe and healthy, just like me.

This person wishes to be happy, just like me.

This person wishes to be loved, just like me.

Now, allow some wishes for wellbeing to arise:

wish that this person have the strength, resources, and social support to navigate the difficulties in life with ease.

I wish that this person be free from pain and suffering.

I wish that this person be peaceful and happy.

I wish that this person be loved.

Because this person is a fellow human being, just like me.

After a few moments, thank your partner with a bow or in whatever way feels appropriate.

References

Chapter 1 – Why Relationships Matter

Ainsworth MD (1969) Object relations, dependency, and attachment: a theoretical review of the infant-mother relationship. Child Development 40 (4):969–1025

Ainsworth MDS, Blehar MC, Waters E, Wall S (1978) Patterns of attachment: A psychological study of the strange situation. Earlbaum, Hillsdale NJ

Bakermans-Krananburg MJ, van IJzendoorn MH, Juffer F (2008) Earlier is better: A meta-analysis of 70 years of intervention improving cognitive development in institutionalized children. Monographs of the Society for Research in Child Development 73(3):279–293

Bartholomew K, Horowitz LM (1991) Attachment styles among young adults: A test of a four-category model. Journal of Personality and Social Psychology 61(2):226–44

Berkman LF, Syme SL (1979) Social networks, host resistance, and mortality: A nine-year follow-up study of Alameda County residents. American Journal of Epidemiology 109(2):186–204

Berlin LJ, Cassidy J, Appleyard K (2008) The influence of early attachments on other relationships. In Cassidy J, Shaver PR (eds) Handbook of attachment: Theory, research and clinical applications. The Guilford Press, New York NY, pp. 333–47

Berlin LJ, Zeanah CH, Lieberman AF (2008) Prevention and intervention programs for supporting early attachment security. In Cassidy J, Shaver PR (eds) Handbook of attachment: Theory, research and clinical applications. The Guilford Press, New York NY, pp. 745–61

Birditt K, Antonucci TC (2008) Life sustaining irritations? Relationship quality and mortality in the context of chronic illness. Social Science & Medicine 67(8):1291–1299

Boden-Albala B, Litwak E, Elkind MS, Rundek T, Sacco RL (2005) Social isolation and outcomes post stroke. Neurology 64(1):1888–92

Bowlby JA (1980) Attachment and loss, volume III: Sadness and depression. Basic Books, New York NY

Bowlby JA (1998) Secure base: Parent–child attachment and healthy human development. Basic Books, New York NY

Bullock BM, Dishion TJ (2007) Family processes and adolescent problem behavior: Integrating relationship narratives into understanding development and change. Journal of the American Academy of Child and Adolescent Psychiatry 46:396–407

Buber M (1971) I and thou, 1st edn. Touchstone, New York NY

Cobb S (1976) Social support as a moderator of life stress. Psychosomatic Medicine 38(5):300–314

Cohen S, Willis TA (1985) Stress, social support, and the buffering hypothesis. Psychological Bulletin 98(2):310–357

Cohen S (2004) Social relationships and health. American Psychologist 59(8):676–684

Cozolino L (2014) The neuroscience of human relationships: Attachment and the developing social brain, 2nd edn. WW Norton & Company Inc., New York NY

Dutton JE (2003) Energize your workplace: How to build and sustain high-quality connections at work. Jossey-Bass Publishers, San Francisco CA

Eaker ED, Sullivan LM, Kelly-Hayes M, D'Agostino RB, Benjamin EJ (2007) Marital status, marital strain, and the risk of coronary heart disease or total mortality: The Framingham offspring study. Psychosomatic Medicine 69:509–513

Eisenberger NI, Taylor SE, Gable SL, Hilmert CJ, Lieberman MD (2007) Neural pathways link social support to attenuated neuroendocrine stress responses. Neuroimage 35:1601–2

Ertel KA, Glymour M, Berkman LF (2009) Social networks and health: a life course perspective integrating observational and experimental evidence. Journal of Social and Personal Relationships 26:73–92

Everson-Rose SA, Lewis TT (2005) Psychosocial factors and cardiovascular diseases. Annual Review of Public Health 26:469–500

Feeny BC, Collins NL (2015) A new look at social support: a theoretical perspective on thriving through relationships. Personality and Social Psychology Review 19(2):113–147

Gleason MEJ, Iida M, Bolger N, Shrout PE (2003) Daily supportive equity in close relationships. Personality Social Psychology Bulletin 29:1036–45

Harlow HF (1959) Love in infant monkeys. Scientific American 200(6):68–74

Haslam SA, Jetten J, Postmes T, Haslam C (2009) Social identity, health and well-being: An emerging agenda for applied psychology. Applied Psychology: An International Review 58(1):1–23

Hawton A (2010) The impact of social isolation on the health status and health-related quality of life of older people. Quality of Life Research 20(1):57–67

Hazan C, Shaver PR (1987) Romantic love conceptualized as an attachment process. Journal of Personality and Social Psychology 52(3):511–24

Hazan C, Shaver PR (1990) Love and work: An attachment theoretical perspective. Journal of Personality and Social Psychology 59(2):270–80

Hazan C, Shaver PR (1994) Attachment as an organizational framework for research on close relationships. Psychological Inquiry 5:1–22

Heaphy ED, Dutton JE (2008) Positive social interactions and the human body at work: Linking organizations and physiology. Academy of Management Review 33:137–162

House JS, Landis KR, Umberson D (1988) Social relationships and health. Science 241:540–5

Holt-Lunstad J, Smith TB, Layton JB (2010) Social relationships and mortality risk: a meta-analytic review. PLoS Med 7:e1000316

Karney BR, Bradbury TN (1995) The longitudinal course of marital quality and stability: A review of theory, method and research. Psychological Bulletin 118(1): 3–34

Kiecolt-Glaser JK (1999) Stress, personal relationships, and immune function: Health implications. Brain, Behavior, and Immunity 13:61–72

Krause N, Goldenhar L, Liang J, Jay G, Maeda D (1993) Stress and exercise among the Japanese elderly. Social Science & Medicine 36:1429–1441

Lazarus RS, Folkman S (1984) Stress, appraisal, and coping. Springer Publishing Company, New York NY

Lewis MA, Rook KS (1999) Social control in personal relationships: Impact on health behaviors and psychological distress. Health Psychology 18:63–71

Lyons-Ruth K, Bureau J-F, Easterbrooks MA, Obsuth I, Hennighausen K, Vulliez-Coady L (2013) Parsing the construct of maternal insensitivity: distinct longitudinal pathways associated with early maternal withdrawal. Attachment & Human Development 15(5–6):562–582

Marcovitch J (1994) Failure to thrive. British Medical Journal 308:35–38

Pearce JW, Pezzot-Pearce TD (2007) Psychotherapy of abused and neglected children, 2nd edn. The Guildford Press, New York NY, pp. 17–20

Poland HJ, Ward MJ (1994) Role of the mother's touch in failure to thrive: A preliminary investigation. Journal of American Academy of Child and Adolescent Psychiatry 33(8):1098–1105

Quinn RW (2007) Energizing others in work relationships. In Dutton JE, Ragins BR (eds) Exploring positive relationships at work: Building a theoretical and research foundation. Routledge, New York NY, pp. 73–90

Robles TF, Kiecolt-Glaser JK (2003) The physiology of marriage: pathways to health. Physiology and Behavior 79:409–16

Selye H (1956) The stress of life. McGraw-Hill Book Co., New York NY

Tucker DM, Luu P, Poulson C (2006) The neurodevelopment process of self-organization. In Cicchetti D (ed) Developmental psychopathology, 3rd edn. John Wiley & Sons, Hoboken NJ

Uchino BN (2006) Social support and health: a review of physiological processes potentially underlying links to disease outcomes. Journal of Behavioral Medicine 29:377–87

Umberson D, Crosnoe R, Reczek C (2010) Social relationships and health behaviors across the life course. Annual Review of Sociology 36:139–57

Wills TA (1991) Social support and interpersonal relationships. In Clark MS (ed) Prosocial behavior. Sage, Newbury Park CA, pp. 265–89

Chapter 2 – Understanding Stress

Beauchaine T (2001) Vagal tone, development, and Gray's motivational theory: toward an integrated model of autonomic nervous system functioning in psychopathology. Development and Psychopathology 13:183–214

Benson H (2000) The relaxation response. Harper Torch, New York NY

Berntson GG, Sarter M, Cacioppo JT (2003) Ascending visceral regulation of cortical affective information processing. European Journal of Neuroscience 18:2103–2109

Brown RP, Gerbarg PL (2009) Yoga breathing, meditation, and longevity. Annals of New York Academic Science 1172:54–62

Brown RP, Gerbarg PL (2012) The healing power of the breath: Simple techniques to reduce stress and anxiety, enhance concentration, and balance your emotions. Shambhala Publications Inc., Boston MA

Boudarene M, Legros JJ, Tilsit-Berthier M (2001) Study of the stress response: role of anxiety, cortisol, and DHEAs. L'encephala 28(2):139–146

Cohen S, Kamarck T, Mermelstein R (1983) A global measure of perceived stress. Journal of Health and Social Behavior 24:386–396

Darwin C (1872) The expression of emotions in man and animals. D Appleton & Company, New York NY, pp. 69

De Couck M, Gidron Y (2013) Norms of vagal nerve activity, indexed by Heart Rate Variability, in cancer patients. Cancer Epidemiology 37:737–741

De Couck M, Mravec B, Gidron Y (2012) You may need the vagus nerve to understand pathophysiology and to treat diseases. Clinical Science (London) 122:323–8

Everly GS Jr, Lating JM (2013) The anatomy and physiology of the human stress response. In Everly GS Jr & Eating JM (eds) A clinical guide to the treatment of the human stress response. Springer, New York NY, pp. 17–21

Gazzaniga MS, Ivry RB, Mangun GR (2013) Cognitive neuroscience: the biology of the mind, 4th edn. WW Norton & Company, New York NY

Gerbarg PL, Brown RP (2015) Yoga and neuronal pathways to enhance stress response, emotion regulation, bonding and spirituality. In Horovitz EG, Elgelid S (eds) Yoga therapy theory and practice. Routledge, New York NY

Gidron Y, De Couck M, De Greve J (2014) If you have an active vagal nerve, cancer stage may no longer be important. Journal of Biologic and Regulatory Homeostatic Agents 28(2): 195–201

Goleman D (2005) Emotional intelligence: Why it can matter more than IQ. Bantam Books, New York NY

Gottman JM, Coan J, Carrere S, Swanson C (1998) Predicting marital happiness and stability from newlywed interactions. Journal of Marriage and the Family 60:5–22

Gottman JM, Silver N (1999) The seven principles for making marriage work: A practical guide from the country's foremost relationship expert. Three Rivers Press, New York NY

Kok BE, Fredrickson BL (2010) Upward spirals of the heart: autonomic flexibility, as indexed by vagal tone, reciprocally and prospectively predicts positive emotions and social connectedness. Biological Psychology 85:432–436

Lazarus RS, Folkman S (1984) Stress, appraisal, and coping. Springer Publishing Company, New York NY

Llewellyn-Smith IJ, Verberne AJM (2011) Central regulation of autonomic functions 2nd Ed. Oxford University Press

Porges SW (1992) Vagal tone: a physiological marker of stress vulnerability. Pediatrics 90:498–504

Porges SW (1996) Physiological regulation in high-risk infants: a model for assessment and potential intervention. Development and Psychopathology 8:43–58

Porges SW (2001) The polyvagal theory: Phylogenetic substrates of a social nervous system. International Journal of Psychophysiology 42:123–146

Porges SW (2009) The polyvagal theory: new insights into adaptive reactions of the autonomic nervous system. Cleveland Clinic Journal of Medicine 76(Suppl. 2):S86–S90

Porges SW (2011) Polyvagal Theory. The neurophysiological foundations of emotions, attachment, communication, and self-regulation. WW Norton & Company, New York NY

Porges SW, Doussard-Roosevelt JA, Maiti AK (1994) Vagal tone and the physiological regulation of emotion. Monographs of the Society for Research in Child Development 59(2–3): 167–186

Porges SW, Doussard-Roosevelt JA, Portales AL, Greenspan SI (1996) Infant regulation of the vagal "brake" predicts child behavior problems: A psychobiological model of social behavior. Developmental Psychobiology 29:697–712

Selye H (1956) The stress of life. McGraw-Hill Book Co., New York NY

Smeets T (2010) Autonomic and hypothalamic-pituitary-adrenal stress resilience: Impact of cardiac vagal tone. Biological Psychology 84(2):290–295

Tsuji H, Larson MG, Venditti FJ, Manders ES, Evans JC, Feldman CL, Levy D (1996) Impact of reduced heart rate variability on risk for cardiac events. Circulation 94:2850–2855

Yuan H, Silberstein, SD (2015a) Vagus nerve and vagus nerve stimulation, a comprehensive review: Part I. Headache 56(1):71–78

Yuan H, Silberstein SD (2015b) Vagus nerve and vagus nerve stimulation, a comprehensive review: Part II. Headache 56(2):259–266

Yuan H, Silberstein SD (2016) Vagus nerve and vagus nerve stimulation, a comprehensive review: Part III. Headache 56(3):479–90

Chapter 3 – Why Manage Chronic Stress?

Arnstein AFT (1999) Development of the cerebral cortex: XIV. Stress impairs prefrontal cortical function. Journal of the American Academy of Child and Adolescent Psychiatry 38(2):219–222

Arnstein AFT (2016) Stress signaling pathways that impair prefrontal cortex structure and function. Nature Reviews Neuroscience 10:410–422

Bremner JD (2005) Does stress damage the brain? Understanding trauma-related disorders from a mind–body perspective. WW Norton & Company, New York NY

Dweck C (2007) Mindset: The new psychology of success. Ballantine Books, New York NY

Everly GS Jr, Lating JM (2013) The anatomy and physiology of the human stress response. In Everly GS Jr & Eating JM (eds) A clinical guide to the treatment of the human stress response. Springer, New York NY, pp. 17–21

Greenberg MS, Taney K, Marin M, Pitman RK (2014) Stress, PTSD, and dementia. Alzheimer's & Dementia 10(3):S155–S165

Gunnar M, Quevedo K (2007) The neurobiology of stress. Annual Review of Psychology 58:145–173

Johansson L, Guo X, Waern M, Östling S, Gustafson D, Bengtsson C, Skoog I (2010) Midlife psychological stress and risk of dementia: a 35-year longitudinal population study. Brain 2217–2224

Karatsoreos IN, McEwen BS (2013) Annual research review: The neurobiology and physiology of resilience and adaptation across the life course. The Journal of Child Psychology and Psychiatry 54(4):337–347

Kemeny ME (2003) The psychobiology of stress. Current Directions in Psychological Science 12(4):124–129

Kendler KS, Karkowski LM, Prescott CA (1999) Causal relationship between stressful life events and the onset of major depression. American Journal of Psychiatry 156:837–841

Killingsworth MA, Gilbert DT (2010) A wandering mind is an unhappy mind. Science 330:932

Lazarus RS (1999) Hope: An emotion and a vital coping resource against despair. Social Research: An International Quarterly 66(2):653–678

Logan JG, Barksdale DJ (2008) Allostasis and allostatic load: Expanding the discourse on stress and cardiovascular disease. Journal of Nursing and Healthcare of Chronic Illness, Journal of Clinical Nursing 17(7b):201–208

Lupien SJ, McEwen BS, Gunnar MR, Heim C (2009) Effects of stress throughout the lifespan on the brain, behavior and cognition. Nature 10:433–445

Mah L, Szabuniewicz C, Fiocco AJ (2016) Can anxiety damage the brain? Current Opinion in Psychiatry 29(1):56

McCormick CM, Mathews IZ (2007) HPA function in adolescence: role of sex hormones in its regulation and the enduring consequences of exposure to stressors. Pharmacology, Biochemistry and Behavior 86:220–233

McEwen BS (1998) Stress, adaptation and disease. Allostasis and allostatic load. Annals of the New York Academy of Sciences 840(1):33–44

McEwen BS (2000) Allostasis and allostatic load: implications for neuropsychopharmacology. Neuropsychopharmacology 22:108–124

Neff LA, Karney BR (2009) Stress and reactivity to daily relationship experiences: How stress hinders adaptive processes in marriage. Journal of Personality and Social Psychology 97(3):435–450

Persson G, Skoog I (1996) A prospective population study of psychosocial risk factors for late onset dementia. International Journal of Geriatric Psychiatry 11:15–22

Roozendaal B, McEwen BS, Chattarji S (2009) Stress, memory, and the amygdala. Nature Reviews, Neuroscience: 10:423–433

Sapolsky RM (1998) Why zebras don't get ulcers: An updated guide to stress-related disease and coping, 2nd edn. WH Freeman, London UK

Schneiderin N, Ironson G, Siegel SD (2005) Stress and health: psychological, behavioral, and biological determinants. Annual Review of Clinical Psychology 1:607–628

Semmer NK, McGrath JE, Beehr TA (2005) Conceptual issues in research on stress and health. In Cooper CL (ed), Handbook of Stress and Health, 2nd edn. CRC Press, New York NY, pp. 1–43

Selye H (1956) The stress of life. McGraw-Hill Book Co., New York NY

Shaw BA, Krause N (2002) The impact of salient role stress on trajectories of health in late life among survivors of a seven-year panel study: analysis of individual growth curves. International Journal on Aging and Human Development 55(2):97–116

Stawski RS, Sliwinsky MJ, Smyth JM, Syracuse University (2006) Stress-related cognitive interference predicts cognitive function in old age. Psychology and Aging 21(3):535–544

Sterling P, Eyer J (1988) Allostasis: A new paradigm to explain arousal pathology. In Fisher S, Reasons J (eds) Handbook of Life Stress, Cognition, and Health. John Wiley & Sons, New York NY, pp. 629–649

Yehuda R, Golier JA, Harvey PD, Stavitsky K, Kaufman S, Grossman RA, Tischler L (2005) Relationship between cortisol and age-related memory impairments in Holocaust survivors with PTSD. Psychoneuroendocrinology 30:678–87

Chapter 4 – The Stories We Tell: Why Mindset Matters

Bandura A, Walters R (1963) Social learning and personality development. Holt, Rinehart, & Winston, New York NY

Bandura A (1977) Social learning theory. General Learning Press, New York NY

Bisby JA, Horner AJ, Horlyck LD, Burgess H (2016) Opposing effects of negative emotion on amygdalar and hippocampal memory for items and associations. Social Cognition Affective Neuroscience 11(6):981–90

Boroditsky L (2011) How language shapes thought. The languages we speak affect our perceptions of the world. Scientific American February:63–65

Bullock BM, Asarnow JR (1998) The association between youth perceptions of their parents and increased risk for youth depression. Poster presentation at University of California, Psychology Undergraduate Research Conference, Los Angeles CA

Bullock BM, Dishion TJ (2004) Family affective attitude rating scale (FAARS). Available from Dr. BG Bullock: bgracebullock@me.com

Bullock BM, Dishion TJ (2007) Family processes and adolescent problem behavior: Integrating relationship narratives into understanding development and change. Journal of the American Academy of Child and Adolescent Psychiatry 46:396–407

Bullock BM, Dishion TJ, Gardner F, Shaw D (2005) Advances in process research: Linking negative affective attitudes, family dynamics, and child and adolescent outcomes. In Bullock B (Chair), *The etiology of children's behavior problems for infancy to middle childhood: Family member attitudes, parenting strategies, and interpersonal processes.* Paper presented at the biennial meeting of the Society for Research in Child Development, Atlanta, GA

Bullock BM, Schneiger A, Dishion TJ (2005) Manual for coding five-minute speech samples using the Family Affective Attitude Rating Scale (FAARS). Available from Dr. BG Bullock: bgracebullock@me.com

Chan D, Woollacott M (2007) Effects of level of meditation experience on attentional focus: Is the efficiency of executive or orientation networks improved? The Journal of Alternative and Complementary Medicine 13(6):651–657

Cohen GL, Sherman DK (2014) The psychology of change: self-affirmation and social psychological intervention. Annual Review of Psychology 65:333–371

Cooley CH (1998) On self and social organization. Schubert H-J (ed) University of Chicago Press, Chicago IL

Fiske ST (1980) Attention and weight in person perception: The impact of negative and extreme behavior. Journal of Personality and Social Psychology 38:889–906

Hayes SC, Blackledge JT, Barnes-Holmes D (2001) Language and cognition: Constructing an alternative approach within the behavioral tradition. In Hayes SC, Barnes-Holmes D, Roche B (eds) Relational frame theory: A post-Skinnerian account of human language and cognition. Kluwer Academic/Plenum, New York NY, pp. 3–20

Hofmann SG, Sawyer AT, Witt, AA, Oh D (2010) The effect of mindfulness-based therapy on anxiety and depression: a meta-analytic review. Journal of Consulting and Clinical Psychology 78(2):169–183

Holtgraves TJ, Kashima Y (2008) Language, meaning, and social cognition. Personality and Social Psychology Review 12:73–94

Konner M (2011) The evolution of childhood: Relationships, emotion, mind. Belknap Press, Cambridge MA

Maslow A (1966) The psychology of science: A reconnaissance. Maurice Bassett Publishing, Chapel Hill NC, p. 15

Moore A, Malinowski P (2009) Meditation, mindfulness, and cognitive flexibility. Consciousness and Cognition 18(1):176–186

Manstead ASR, Fischer AH (2001) The social world as object of and influence on appraisal processes. In Scherer KR, Schorr A, Johnstone T (eds) Appraisal processes in emotion: theory, methods, research. Oxford University Press, Oxford UK, pp. 221–232

Öhman A, Mineka S (2001) Fears, phobias, and preparedness: Toward an evolved module of fear and fear learning. Psychological Review 108:483–522

Pasalich DS, Dadds MR, Hawes DJ, Brennan J (2011) Assessing relational schemas in parents of children with externalizing behavior disorders: reliability and validity of the family affective attitude rating scale. Psychiatry Research 185:438–443

Pennebaker JW, Mehl MR, Niederhoffer KG (2003) Psychological aspects of natural language use: Our words, our selves. Annual Review of Psychology 54:547–577

Piaget J (1936) Origins of intelligence in the child. Routledge & Kegan Paul, London UK

Plous S (1993) The psychology of judgment and decision making. McGraw-Hill Book Co., New York NY

Singer MA (2007) The untethered soul. New Harbinger Publications, Oakland CA

Smith JD, Dishion T, Moore KJ, Shaw DS, Wilson MN (2013) Effects of video feedback on early coercive parent–child interactions: The intervening role of caregiver's relational schemas. Journal of Clinical Child and Adolescent Psychology 42(3):405–417

Taylor SE (1991) Asymmetrical effects of positive and negative events: the mobilization-minimization hypothesis. Psychological Bulletin 110(1):67–85

Vaish A, Grossman T, Woodward A (2008) Not all emotions are created equal: The negativity bias in social-emotional development. Psychology Bulletin 134(3):383–403

Waller R, Gardner F, Dishion TJ, Shaw DS, Wilson M (2012) Validity of a brief measure of parental affective attitudes in high-risk preschoolers. Journal of Abnormal Child Psychology 40(6):945–955

Chapter 5 – Mindfulness and The Mind

Arnstein AFT (1999) Development of the cerebral cortex: XIV. Stress impairs prefrontal cortical function. Journal of American Academy of Child and Adolescent Psychiatry 38(2):220–222

Arnstein AFT (2009) Stress signaling pathways that impair prefrontal cortex structure and function. Nature Reviews Neuroscience 10:410–422

Baer RA (2003) Mindfulness training as a clinical intervention: A conceptual and empirical review. Clinical Psychology: Science and Practice 10(2):125–143

Barnes S, Brown KW, Krusemark E, Campbell WK, Rogge RD (2007) The role of mindfulness in romantic relationship satisfaction and responses to relationship stress. Journal of Marital and Family Therapy 33(4):482–500

Boccia M, Piccardi L, Guariglia P (2015) The meditative mind: A comprehensive meta-analysis of MRI studies. BioMed Research International 2015:419808

Brewer JA, Worhunsky PD, Gray J, Tang Y, Weber J, Kober H (2011) Meditation experience is associated with differences in default mode network activity and connectivity. PNAS 108(50):20254–20259

Brown KW, Ryan RM (2003) The benefits of being present: Mindfulness and its role in psychological wellbeing. Journal of Personality and Social Psychology 84(4):822–848

Brown KW, Ryan RM, Creswell JD (2007) Mindfulness: theoretical foundations and evidence for its salutary effects. Psychological Inquiry 18:211–237

Buckner RL, Andrews-Hanna JR, Schacter DL (2008) The brain's default network: anatomy, function, and relevance to disease. Annals of the New York Academy of Sciences 1124(1):1–38

Burpee LC, Langer EJ (2005) Mindfulness and marital satisfaction. Journal of Adult Development 12(1):43–51

Carson JW, Carson KM, Gil KM, Baucom DH (2004) Mindfulness-based relationship enhancement. Behavior Therapy 35(3):471–494

Cherkin DC, Sherman KJ, Balderson BH, Cook AJ, Anderson ML, Hawkes RJ, Hansen KE, Turner JA (2016) Effect of mindfulness-based stress reduction vs cognitive-behavioral therapy of usual care on back pain and functional limitations in adults with chronic low back pain: A randomized clinical trial. Journal of the American Medical Association 315(12):1240–1249

Chisea A, Serretti A (2009) Mindfulness-based stress reduction for stress management in healthy people: a review and meta-analysis. The Journal of Complementary and Alternative Medicine 15(5):593–600

Clarke TC, Black LI, Stussman BJ, Barnes PM, Nahin RL (2015) Trends in the use of complementary health approaches among adults: United States 2002–2012. National Health Statistics Reports 79:February 10

Coronado-Montoya S, Levis AW, Kwakkenbos L, Steele RJ, Turner EH, Thombs BD (2016) Reporting of positive results in randomized controlled trials of mindfulness-based mental health interventions. PLoS ONE 11(4):e0153220

Creswell JD, Myers HF, Cole SW, Irwin MR (2009) Mindfulness meditation training effects on CD4+ T lymphocytes in HIV-1 infected adults: A small randomized controlled trial. Brain, Behavior, and Immunity 23:184–188

Creswell JD, Taren AA, Lindsay EK, Greco CM, Gianaros PJ, Fairgrieve A, Marsland AL, Brown KW, Way BM, Rosen RK, Ferris JL (2016) Alterations in resting state functional connectivity link mindfulness meditation with reduced interleukin-6: a randomized controlled trial. Biological Psychiatry 80(1):53–61

Davidson RJ, Kabat-Zinn J, Schumacher J, Rosenkranz M, Muller D, Santorelli SF, Urbanowski F, Harrington A, Bonus K, Sheridan JF (2003) Alterations in brain and immune function produced by mindfulness meditation. Psychosomatic Medicine 65:564–570

Davis DM, Hayes JA (2011) What are the benefits of mindfulness? A practice review of psychotherapy-related research. Psychotherapy 48(2):198–208

Desbordes G, Negó LT, Pace TWW, Wallace BA, Raison CL, Schwartz EL (2012) Effects of mindful-attention and compassion meditation training on amygdala response to emotional stimuli in an ordinary, non-meditative state. Frontiers in Human Neuroscience 6(292):1–15

Farb NA, Anderson AK, Mayberg H, Bean J, McKeon D, Segal ZV (2010) Minding one's emotions: mindfulness training alters the neural expression of sadness. Emotion 10:25–33

Farias M, Wilkholm C (2015) The Buddha pill: Can meditation change you? Watkins Publishing, London UK

Fox KCR, Nijeboer V, Dixon JL, Floman JL, Ellamiil M, Rumak SP, Sedlmeier P, Christoff K (2014) Is meditation associated with altered brain structure? A systematic review and meta-analysis of morphometric neuroimaging in meditation practitioners. Neuroscience & Biobehavioral Reviews 43:48–73

Gard T, Noggle JJ, Park CL, Vago DR, Wilson A (2014) Potential self-regulatory mechanisms of yoga for psychological health. Frontiers in Human Neuroscience 8(770):1–20

Garrison KA, Zeffiro TA, Scheinost D, Constable RT, Brewer JA (2015) Meditation leads to reduced default mode network activity beyond an active task. Cognitive, Affective, & Behavioral Neuroscience 15:712–720

Gambrel LE, Piercy FP (2014a) Mindfulness-based relationship education for couples expecting their first child – Part 1: A randomized mixed-methods program evaluation. Journal of Marital and Family Therapy 41(1):5–24

Gambrel LE, Piercy FP (2014b) Mindfulness-based relationship education for couples expecting their first child – Part 2: Phenomenological findings. Journal of Marital and Family Therapy 41(1):25–41

Gelles D (2015) Mindful work: How meditation is changing business from the inside out. Houghton Mifflin Harcourt, New York NY

Goldin PR, Gross JJ (2010) Effects of mindfulness-based stress reduction (MBSR) on emotion regulation in social anxiety disorder. Emotion 10:83–91

Goyal M, Singh S, Sibinga EM, Gould NF, Rowland-Seymour A, Sharma R, Berger Z, Sleicher D, Maron DD, Shihab HM, Ranasinghe PD, Linn S, Saha S, Bass EB, Haythornthwaite JA (2014) Meditation programs for psychological stress and well-being: a systematic review and meta-analysis. Journal of the American Medical Association Intern Medicine 174:357–368

Grossman P, Niemann L, Schmidt S, Walach H (2004) Mindfulness-based stress reduction and health benefits. A meta-analysis. Journal of Psychosomatic Research 57:35–42

Grossman P, Tiefenthaler-Gilmer U, Raysz A, Kesper U (2007) Mindfulness training as an intervention for fibromyalgia: Evidence of postintervention and three-year follow-up benefits in wellbeing. Psychotherapy and Psychosomatics 76:226–233

Hayes SC, Strosahl KD, Wilson KG (1999) Acceptance and commitment therapy: An experiential approach to behavior change. The Guilford Press, New York NY

Hofmann SG, Sawyer AT, Witt AA, Oh D (2010) The effect of mindfulness-based therapy on anxiety and depression: A meta-analytic review. Journal of Consulting and Clinical Psychology 78, 169–183

Hölzel BK, Carmody J, Evans KC, Hoge EA, Dusek JA, Morgan L, Pitman RK, Lazar SW (2010) Stress reduction correlates with structural changes in the amygdala. Social Cognitive and Affective Neuroscience 5(1):11–17

Hölzel BK, Carmody J, Vangel M, Congleton C, Yerramsetti SM, Gard T, Lazar SW (2011a) Mindfulness practice leads to increases in regional brain gray matter density. Psychiatry Research 191(1):36–43

Hölzel BK, Lazar SW, Gard T, Schuman-Olivier Z, Vago DR, Ott U (2011b) How does mindfulness meditation work? Proposing mechanisms of action from a conceptual and neural perspective. Perspectives on Psychological Science 6(6):537–559

Jacobson NS, Christensen A (1996) Integrative couples therapy: Promoting acceptance and change. Norton, New York NY

Jang JH, Jung WH, Kang D, Byun MS, Kwon SJ, Choi CH, Kwon JS (2011) Increased default mode network connectivity associated with meditation. Neuroscience letters 487(3):358–362

Jha AP, Krompinger J, Baime MJ (2007) Mindfulness training modifies subsystems of attention. Cognitive Affective Behavioral Neuroscience 7:109–119

Kabat-Zinn J (1990) Full catastrophe living: Using the wisdom of your body and mind to face stress, pain, and illness. Delacorte, New York NY

Khoury B, Lecomte T, Fortin G, Masse M, Therien P, Bouchard V, Chapleau MA, Paquin K, Hofmann SG (2013) Mindfulness-based therapy: a comprehensive meta-analysis. Clinical Psychology Review 33(6):763–771

Khoury B, Sharma M, Rush SE, Fournier C (2015) Mindfulness-based stress reduction for healthy individuals: A meta-analysis. Journal of Psychosomatic Research 78(6):519–528

Kozlowski A (2013) Mindful mating: Exploring the connection between mindfulness and relationship satisfaction. Sexual and Relationship Therapy 28(1–2):92–104

Lazar SW, Kerr CE, Wasserman RH, Gray JR, Greve DN, Treadway MT, McGarvey M, Quinn BT, Dusek JA, Benson H, Rauch SL, Moore CI, Fischl B (2005) Meditation experience is associated with increased cortical thickness. Neuroreport 16(17):1893–1897

Linehan MM (1993) Cognitive-behavioral treatment of borderline personality disorder. The Guilford Press, New York NY

Lutz A, Brefczynski-Lewis J, Johnstone T, Davidson RJ (2008) Regulation of the neural circuitry of emotion by compassion meditation: effects of meditative expertise. PLoS ONE 3:e1897

Lutz A, Slager HA, Rawlings NB, Francis AD, Greischar LL, Davidson RJ (2009) Mental training enhances attentional stability: Neural and behavioral evidence. Journal of Neuroscience 29:13418–13427

McGill J, Adler-Baeder F, Rodriguez P (2016) Mindfully in love: A meta-analysis of the association between mindfulness and relationship satisfaction. Journal of Human Sciences and Extension 4(1):89–101

Moore A, Gruber T, Derose J, Malinowski P (2012) Regular, brief mindfulness meditation practice improves electrophysiological markers of attentional control. Frontiers in Human Neuroscience 6:18

Pascoe MC, Bauer IE (2015) A systematic review of randomized control trials on the effects of yoga on stress measures and mood. Journal of Psychiatric Research 68:270–282

Segal ZV, Teasdale JD, Williams JMG (2004) Mindfulness-based cognitive therapy: Theoretical rationale and empirical status. In Hayes SC, Follette VM, Linehan MM (eds) Mindfulness and relationship: Expanding the cognitive behavioral relationship. The Guilford Press, New York NY, pp. 45–65

Segal ZV, Bieling P, Young T, MacQueen G, Cooke R, Martin L, Bloch R, Levitan RD (2010) Antidepressant monotherapy vs sequential pharmacotherapy and mindfulness-based cognitive therapy, or placebo, for relapse prophylaxis in recurrent depression. Archives of General Psychiatry 67:1256

Sharf RH (2015) Is mindfulness Buddhist? (And why it matters). Transcultural Psychiatry 52(4):470–484

Shatz C (1992) The developing brain. Scientific American 267(3):60–67

Simpkins A, Simpkins AM (2013) Neuroscience for clinicians: Evidences, models, and practice. Springer, New York NY

Streeter CC, Whitfield TH, Owen L, Rein T, Karri SK, Yakhkind A, Perlmutter R, Prescot A, Renshaw PF, Ciraulo DA, Jensen JE (2010) Effects of yoga versus walking on mood, anxiety, and brain GABA levels: A randomized controlled MRS study. The Journal of Complementary and Alternative Medicine 16(11):1145–1152

Streeter CC, Gerberg PL, Saper RB, Ciraulo DA, Brown RP (2012) Effects of yoga on the autonomic nervous system, gamma-aminobutyric-acid, and allostasis in epilepsy, depression, and post-traumatic stress disorder. Medical Hypotheses 78(5):571–579

Sykes Wylie M (2015) How the mindfulness movement went mainstream – and the backlash that came with it. Psychotherapy Networker, Alternet [Online] Available at: http://www.alternet.org/personal-health/how-mindfulness-movement-went-mainstream-and-backlash-came-it

Tang Y-Y, Hölzel BK, Posner MI (2015) The neuroscience of mindfulness meditation. Nature Reviews Neuroscience 16:213–225

Tapper K, Shaw C, Ilsley J, Hill AJ, Bond FW, Moore L (2009) Exploratory randomized controlled trial of a mindfulness-based weight loss intervention for women. Appetite 52:396–404

Teasdale JD, Segal ZV, Mark J, Ridgeway VA, Soulsby JM, Lau MA (2000) Prevention of relapse/recurrence in major depression by mindfulness-based cognitive therapy. Journal of Consulting and Clinical Psychology 68:615–623

Telles S, Raghavendra BR, Naveen K, Manjunath N, Kumar S, Subramanya P (2013) Changes in autonomic variables following two meditative states described in yoga texts. The Journal of Alternative and Complementary Medicine 19(1):35–42

Tomasino B, Fregona S, Skrap M, Fabbro F (2013) Meditation related activations are modulated by the practices needed to obtain it and by the expertise: An ALE meta-analysis study. Frontiers in Human Neuroscience 6:346

Vago DR, Silbersweig DA (2012) Self-awareness, self-regulation, and self-transcendence (S-ART): A framework for understanding the neurobiological mechanisms of mindfulness. Frontiers in Human Neuroscience 6:296

Wenk-Sormaz H (2005) Meditation can reduce habitual responding. Alternative Therapies 11(2):42–51

Chapter 6 – Personal Responsibility and Social Change

Asch SE (1955) Opinions and social pressure. Scientific American 193(5):31–35

Banaji M, Heiphetz L (2010) Attitudes. In Fiske S, Gilbert D, Lindzey G (eds) Handbook of social psychology, 5th edn. Wiley, New York NY, pp. 348-388

Dervin F (2012) Cultural identity, representation, and bothering. In Jackson J (ed) The Routledge handbook of language and intercultural communication. Routledge, New York NY, pp. 181–194

Devine P (1989) Stereotypes and prejudice: Their automatic and controlled components. Journal of Personality and Social Psychology 56:5–18

Golding W (1962) Lord of the flies. Coward-McCann, New York NY

Greenwald AG, McGhee DE, Schwartz JLK (1998) Measuring the individual differences in implicit cognition: the implicit association test. Journal of Personality and Social Psychology 74(6):1464-1480

Groom B, Bailenson JN, Naas C (2009) The influence of racial embodiment on racial bias in immersive virtual environments. Social Influence iFirst Article:1–18

Haney C, Banks C, Zimbardo P (1973) Interpersonal dynamics in a simulated prison. International Journal of Criminology and Penology 1:69–97

Janis IL (1982) Groupthink, 2nd edn. Houghton Mifflin, Boston MA

Jung CG (1938) Psychology and religion. Yale University Press, Stamford CT

Lieberman MD, Rock D, Cox CL (2014) Breaking bias. Neuroleadership Journal 5

Milgram S (1963) Behavioral study of obedience. Journal of Abnormal Social Psychology 67:371–8

Peck TC, Seinfeld S, Aglioti SM, Slater M (2013) Putting yourself in the skin of a black avatar reduces implicit racial bias. Consciousness and Cognition 22(3):799–787

Peters W (1971) A class divided. Doubleday and Company Inc., New York NY

Phelps EA, O'Connor KJ, Cunningham WA, Funayama ES, Gatenby JC, Gore JC, Banaji MR (2000) Performance on indirect measures of race evaluation predicts amygdala activation. Journal of Cognitive Neuroscience 12(5):729–738

Reynolds EA, Losin R, Cross KA, Iacoboni M, Dapretto M (2014) Neural processing of race during imitation: Self-similarity versus social status. Human Brain Mapping 35:1723–1739

Rudman L (2004) Social justice in our minds, homes, and society: The nature, causes, and consequences of implicit bias. Social Justice Research 17:129–142

Senge P (2006) The fifth discipline: The art & practice of the learning organization, revised edn. Doubleday, New York NY

Sumner WG (1906) Folkways: A study of mores, manners, customs, and morals. Ginn & Company, Boston MA, p. 12

Chapter 7 – The BREATHE Model

Dunkel Schetter C, Dolbier C (2011) Resilience in the context of chronic stress and health in adults. Social and Personality Psychology Compass 5(9):634-652

Elliott S, Edmonson D (2006) The new science of the breath: coherent breathing for autonomic nervous system balance, health and wellbeing. Coherence Press, Allen TX

Iyengar BKS (1995) Light on yoga: yoga dipika. Schocken, New York NY

James W (1884) What is an emotion? Mind 9(34):188–205

Jerath R, Edry JW, Barnes VA, Jerath V (2006) Physiology of long pranayamic breathing: Neural respiratory elements may provide a mechanism that explains how slow deep breathing shifts the autonomic nervous system. Medical Hypothesis 67:566–571

Selye H (1956) The stress of life. McGraw-Hill Book Co., New York NY

Sovik R (2000) The science of breathing – the yogic view. Progress in Brain Research 122:491–505

Chapter 8 – Breath Awareness

Brown RP, Gerbarg PL (2005a) Sudarshan Kriyga Yogic breathing in the treatment of stress, anxiety, and depression: Part I – Neurophysiologic model. The Journal of Alternative and Complementary Medicine 11(1):189–201

Brown RP, Gerbarg PL (2005b) Sudarshan Kriyga Yogic breathing in the treatment of stress, anxiety, and depression: Part II – Clinical applications and guidelines. The Journal of Alternative and Complementary Medicine 11(4):711–717

Brown RP, Gerbarg PL (2012) The healing power of the breath: simple techniques to reduce stress and anxiety, enhance concentration, and balance your emotions. Shambhala Publications Inc., Boston MA

Elliott S, Edmonson D (2006) The new science of the breath: coherent breathing for autonomic nervous system balance, health and wellbeing. Coherence Press, Allen TX

Fried R (1999) Breathe well, be well: A program to relieve stress, anxiety, asthma, hypertension, migraine, and other disorders for better health. John Wiley & Sons, Inc., New York NY

Gottman JM, Silver N (2015) The seven principles for making marriage work: A practical guide from the country's foremost relationship expert. Harmony Books, New York NY

Guz A (1997) Brain, breathing, and breathlessness. Respiration Physiology 109:197–204

Homma I, Masaoka Y (2008) Breathing rhythms and emotions. Experimental Physiology 93(9):1011–1021

Levine PA (1997) Waking the tiger: Healing trauma. North Atlantic Books, Berkeley CA

Sovik R (2000) The science of breathing – The yogic view. Progress in Brain Research 122:491–505

van der Kolk B (2015) The body keeps the score: Brain, mind, and body in the healing of trauma. Viking, New York NY

Chapter 9 – Regulating the Autonomic Nervous System Through Intentional Breathing

Benson H, Beary JF, Carol MP (1974) The relaxation response. Psychiatry 37:37–46

Binello G, Nastri M, Mazzola A, de Lujan Calcagno M, del Luca S, Pueyrredón JH, Salvat F (2016) Yoga therapy longhana breathing practice for chronic pain management. Merit Research Journal of Medicine and Medical Sciences 4(2):79–91

Brown RP, Gerbarg PL (2005a) Sudarshan Kriyga Yogic breathing in the treatment of stress, anxiety, and depression: Part I – Neurophysiologic model. The Journal of Alternative and Complementary Medicine 11(1):189–201

Brown RP, Gerbarg PL (2005b) Sudarshan Kriyga Yogic Breathing in the treatment of stress, anxiety, and depression: Part II – Clinical applications and guidelines. The Journal of Alternative and Complementary Medicine 11(4):711–717

Brown RP, Gerbarg PL (2009) Yoga breathing, meditation, and longevity. Annals of New York Academic Science 1172:54–62

Brown RP, Gerbarg PL (2012) The healing power of the breath: simple techniques to reduce stress and anxiety, enhance concentration, and balance your emotions. Shambhala Publications Inc., Boston MA

Ducla-Soares JL, Santos-Bento M, Laranjo S, Andrade A, Ducla-Soares E, Boto JP, Silva-Carvalho L, Rocha I (2007) Wavelet analysis of autonomic outflow of normal subjects on head-up tilt, cold pressor test, Valsalva maneuver and deep breathing. Experimental Physiology 92(4):677–686

Elliott S, Edmonson D (2006) The new science of the breath: Coherent breathing for autonomic nervous system balance, health and wellbeing. Coherence Press, Allen TX

Fried R (1999) Breathe well, be well: A program to relieve stress, anxiety, asthma, hypertension, migraine, and other disorders for better health. John Wiley & Sons, Inc., New York NY

Homma I, Masaoka Y (2008) Breathing rhythms and emotions. Experimental Physiology 93(9):1011–1021

Iyengar BKS (1985) Light on pranayama: The yogic art of breathing. The Crossroad Publishing Company, New York NY

Iyengar BKS (2004) Astadala yogamala (Collected works), volume 2. Allied Publishers, New Delhi India

Jerath R, Edry JW, Barnes VA, Jerath V (2006) Physiology of long pranayamic breathing: neural respiratory elements may provide a mechanism that explains how slow deep breathing shifts the autonomic nervous system. Medical Hypotheses 67(3):566–571

Ley R (1999) The modification of breathing behavior. Pavlovian and operant control in emotion and cognition. Behavior Modification 23:441–479

Nerurkar A, Yeh G, Davis RB, Birdee G, Phillips RS (2011) When conventional medical providers recommend unconventional medicine: Results of a national study. Archives of Internal Medicine 171(9):862–864

Porges SW (2011) Polyvagal theory. The neurophysiological foundations of emotions, attachment, communication and self-regulation. WW Norton & Company

Rickard KB, Dunn DJ, Brouch VM (2015) Breathing techniques associated with improved health outcomes. Virginia Henderson Global Nursing e-Repository. Retrieved from http://www.nursinglibrary.org/vhl/handle/10755/558648

Sakakibara M, Hayano J (1996) Effect of slowed respiration on cardiac parasympathetic response to threat. Psychosomatic Medicine 58:32–37

Sovik R (2000) The science of breathing – The yogic view. Progress in Brain Research 122:491–505

Telles S, Raghavendra BR, Naveen K, Manjunath N, Kumar S, Subramanya P (2013) Changes in autonomic variables following two meditative states described in yoga texts. The Journal of Alternative and Complementary Medicine 19(1):35–42

Yoshikawa T, Naito Y (2000) What is oxidative stress? Journal of the Japan Medical Association 124(11):1549–1553

Chapter 10 – Experiencing Emotion

Barrett LF, Quigley KS, Bliss-Moreau E, Aronson KR (2004) Interoceptive sensitivity and self-reports of emotional experience. Journal of Personality and Social Psychology 87(5):684–697

Bolte Taylor J (2009) My stroke of insight: A brain scientist's personal journey. Plume, New York NY

Cannon WB (1927) The James-Lange theory of emotion: A critical examination and an alternative theory. American Journal of Psychology 39:106–124

Critchley HD, Wiens S, Rothstein P, Öhman A, Dolan RJ (2004) Neural systems supporting interoceptive awareness. Nature Neuroscience 7(2):189–195

Damasio A (1999) The feeling of what happens: Body and emotion in the making of consciousness. Harcourt, New York NY

Fleet RP, Beitman BD (1998) Cardiovascular death from panic disorder and panic-like anxiety: A critical review of the literature. Journal of Psychosomatic Research 44(1):71–80

Friedman BH, Thayer JF (1998) Autonomic balance revisited: Panic, anxiety and heart rate variability. Journal of Psychosomatic Research 44(1):133–151

Green EE, Green AM, Walters ED (1979) Biofeedback for mind/body self-regulation: Healing and creativity. In Peper E, Anconi S, Quinn M (eds) Mind/body integration: Essential readings in biofeedback. Plenum Press, New York NY

Goleman D (2005) Emotional intelligence: Why it can matter more than IQ, 10th anniversary edn. Bantam Books, New York NY

Haase L, Steward JL, Youssef B, May AC, Isakovic S, Simmons AN, Johnson DC, Potterat EG, Paulus MP (2015) When the brain does not adequately feel the body: Links between low resilience and interoception. Biological Psychology 113:37–45

HeartMath Institute [Online] Available at: http://www.heartmath.org

James W (1884) What is an emotion? Mind 9(34):188–205

Lessmeier TJ, Gamperling D, Johnson-Liddon V, Fromm BS, Steinman RT, Meissner MD, Lehmann MH (1997) Unrecognized paroxysmal supraventricular tachycardia: potential for misdiagnosis as panic disorder. Archives of Internal Medicine 157:537–543

Licht CMM, de Geus EJC, van Dyck R, Penninx BWJH (2009) Association between anxiety disorders and heart rate variability in the Netherlands study of depression and anxiety (NESDA). Psychosomatic Medicine 71:508–518

Mate G (2011) When the body says no: Exploring the stress–disease connection. Wiley, New York NY

McCraty R (2015a) The science of the heart: Exploring the role of the heart in human performance, Volume 2. HeartMath Institute, Boulder Creek CA

McCraty R (2015b) Heart–brain neurodynamics: the making of emotion. In Dalitz M, Hall G (eds) Issues of the Heart: The Neuropsychotherapist special issue 76–110

McCraty R, Atkinson M, Bradley RT (2004) Electrophysiological evidence of intuition: Part 2. A system-wide process? Journal of Alternative and Complementary Medicine 10:325–336

Mossbridge JA, Tressoldi P, Utts J, Ives JA, Radin D, Jonas WB (2014) Predicting the unpredictable: Critical analysis and practical implications of predictive anticipatory activity. Frontiers in Human Neuroscience 8:146

Nummenmaa L, Glerean E, Hari R Heitanen JK (2014) Bodily maps of emotions. Proceedings of the National Academy of Sciences 111(2):646–651

Papez JW (1937) A proposed mechanism of emotion. The Journal of Neuropsychiatry & Clinical Neurosciences 1995 Winter;7(1):103–12

Pollatos O, Gramann K, Schandry R, (2007) Neural systems connecting interoceptive awareness and feelings. Human Brain Mapping 28(1):9–18

Radin D (1997) Unconscious perception of future emotions: an experiment in presentiment. Journal of Scientific Exploration 11:163–180

Schultz A, Vogele C (2015) Interception and stress. Frontiers in Psychology 6:993

Sternberg EM (2001) The balance within: The science connecting health and emotions. WH Freeman, London UK

Terasawa Y, Fukushima H, Umeda S (2013) How does interoceptive awareness interact with the subjective experience of emotion? An fMRI study. Human Brain Mapping 34:598–612

van der Kolk B (2015) The body keeps the score: brain, mind, and body in the healing of trauma. Penguin Books

Wiens S (2005) Interoception in emotional experience. Current Opinion in Neurology 18(4):442–447

Chapter 11 – Appraising and Adjusting Your Mindset

Dweck C (2007) Mindset: The new psychology of success. Ballantine Books, New York NY Folkman S, Lazarus RS, Dunkel-Schetter C, DeLongis A, Gruen R (1986) Dynamics of a stressful encounter: Cognitive appraisal, coping, and encounter outcomes. Journal of Personality and Social Psychology 50(5):992–1003

Folkman S, Lazarus RS, Dunkel-Schetter C, DeLongis A, Gruen R (1986) Dynamics of a stressful encounter: cognitive appraisal, coping, and encounter outcomes. Journal of Personality and Social Psychology 50(5):992-1003

Gorkin, C (2015) "Worst Day Ever?" [Online] Available at: http://www.poetrynation.com/poem.php?id=50509

Gottman JM, Silver N (1999) The seven principles for making marriage work: A practical guide from the country's foremost relationship expert. Three Rivers Press, New York NY

Hammond KR (1999) Judgments under stress. Oxford University Press, Oxford UK

Heider F (1958) The psychology of interpersonal relations. Wiley, New York NY

Kelly HH (1974) The process of causal attribution. American Psychologist 107–128

Lazarus RS, Folkman S (1984) Stress, appraisal, and coping. Springer Publishing Company, New York NY

Maslow AH (1966) Psychology of science. J. Dewey Society: Joanna Cotler Books, New York NY

Nickerson RS (1998) Confirmation bias: A ubiquitous phenomenon in many guises. Review of General Psychology 2(2):175–220

Singer MA (2007) The untethered soul. New Harbinger Publications Inc., Oakland CA

Weiner B (1992) Human motivation: Metaphors, theories, and research. Sage Publications, New York NY

Weiner B (1995) Judgments of responsibility: A foundation for a theory of social conduct. The Guilford Press, New York NY

Chapter 12 – Taking a Purposeful Pause

Ahola K, Hakanen J, Perhoniemi R, Mutanen P (2014) Relationship between burnout and depressive symptoms: a study using the person-centred approach. Burnout Research 1:29-37

Bakker AB, Costa PL (2014) Chronic job burnout and daily functioning: a theoretical analysis. Burnout Research 1:112-119

Benson H, Beary JF, Carol MP (1974) The relaxation response. Psychiatry 37:37–46

Binnewies C, Sonnetag S, Mojza EJ (2010) Recovery during the weekend and fluctuations in weekly job performance: A week-level study examining intra-individual relationships. Journal of Occupational and Organizational Psychology 83(2):419–441

Fisher A (2015) Why don't Americans take more time off? Fortune [Online] Available at: http://fortune.com/2015/07/28/americans-vacation-use/

Gottselig JM, Hofer-Tinguely G, Burley AA, Regel SJ, Lancelot HP, Rétey JV, Achermann P (2004) Sleep and rest facilitate auditory learning. Neuroscience 127:557–561

Groch S, Wilhelm I, Diekelmann S, Born J (2013) The role of REM sleep in the processing of emotional memories: Evidence from behavior and event-related potentials. Neurobiology of Learning and Memory 99:1–9

Haslach C, Schaufelt WB, Leiter MP (2001) Job burnout. Annual Review of Psychology 52:397–422

Innanen H, Tolvanen A, Salmela-Aro K (2014) Burnout, work engagement and workaholism among highly educated employees: profiles, antecedents and outcomes. Burnout Research 1:38-49

Kabat-Zinn J (1994) Wherever you go, there you are. Hyperion, New York NY

Krystal AD (2012) Psychiatric disorders and sleep. Neurology Clinics 30(4):1389–1413

Llorens-Gumbau S, Salanova-Soria M (2014) Loss and gain cycles? A longitudinal study about burnout, engagement and self-efficacy. Burnout Research 1:3-11

Maas JB, Wherry ML, Axelrod DJ, Hogan BR, Blumin J (1998) Power sleep: The revolutionary program that prepares your mind for peak performance. Villard, New York NY

Oppezzo M, Schwartz DL (2014) Give your ideas some legs: The positive effect of walking on creative thinking. Journal of Experimental Psychology; Learning, Memory, and Cognition 40(14):1142–1152

Sonnetag S (2003) Recovery, work engagement, and proactive behavior: A new look at the interface between nonwork and work. Journal of Applied Psychology 88(3):518–528

Sonnetag S, Fritz C (2006) Recovery, wellbeing, and performance-related outcomes: The role of workload and vacation expectancies. Journal of Applied Psychology 91(4):936–945

Sonnentag S, Fritz C (2007) The recovery experience questionnaire: Development and validation of a measure for assessing recuperation and unwinding from work. Journal of Occupational Health Psychology 12:204–221

Sternberg EM (2001) The balance within: the science connecting health and emotions. WH Freeman

Stickgold R, Hobson JA, Fosse R, Fosse M (2001) Sleep, learning, and dreams: Off-line memory reprocessing. Science 294:1052–1057

Chapter 13 – Humor: Life as Practice

Abel MH (1998) Interaction of humor and gender in moderation relationships between stress and outcomes. The Journal of Psychology 132:267–276

Abel MH (2002) Humor, stress, and coping strategies. Humor 15(4):365–381

Brownell HH, Gardner H (1988) Neuropsychological insights into humor. In Durant J, Miller J (eds) Laughing matters: a serious look at humor. Wiley, New York NY, pp. 17–34

Fry WF Jr (1992) The physiologic effects of humor, mirth, and laughter. The Journal of the American Medical Association 267:1857–1858

Labott SM, Ahleman SW, Wolever ME, Martin RB (1990) The physiological and psychological effects of the expression and inhibition of emotion. Behavioral Medicine 16:182–189

Lefcourt HM, Martin RA (1986) Humor and life stress: antidote to adversity. Springer-Verlag, New York NY

Lefcourt HM, Davidson-Katz K, Kueneman K (1990) Humor and immune-system functioning. Humor 3:305–21

Martin RA (2002) Is laughter the best medicine? Humor, laughter, and physical health. Current Directions in Psychological Science 11(6):216–220

Martin RA, Dobbin JP (1988) Sense of humor, hassles, and immunoglobin A: Evidence for a stress-moderating effect. International Journal of Psychiatry in Medicine 18:93–105

Merriam-Webster (2016) The Merriam-Webster dictionary, new edn. Merriam-Webster Inc., Springfield MA

Chapter 14 – Engaging Others Mindfully

Christov-Moore L, Iacoboni M (2016) Self-other resonance, its control and prosocial inclinations: Brain-behavior relationships. Human Brain Mapping 37:1544–1558

Gump BB, Kulik JA (1997) Stress, affiliation, and emotional contagion. Journal of Personality and Social Psychology 72(2):305–319

Hatfield E, Cacioppo JT (1994) Emotional contagion: Studies in emotion and social interaction. Cambridge University Press, Cambridge UK

Iacoboni M (2009) Mirroring people: The science of empathy and how we connect with others. Picador, London UK

Inagaki TK, Bryne Haltom KE, Suzuki S, Jevtic I, Hornstein E, Bower JE, Eisenberger NI (2016) The neurobiology of giving versus receiving support. Psychosomatic Medicine 78(4):443–53

Joiner TE, Katz J (1999) Contagion of depressive symptoms and mood: Meta-analytic review and explanations from cognitive, behavioral, and interpersonal viewpoints. Clinical Psychology: Science and Practice 6(2):149–164

Levy DA, Nail PR (1993) Contagion: A theoretical and empirical review and reconceptualization. Genetic, Social, & General Psychology Monographs 119(2):1–42

McTaggart L (2012) The bond: How to fix your falling-down world. Free Press, New York NY

Parkinson B (2011) Interpersonal emotion transfer: Contagion and social appraisal. Social and Personality Psychology Compass 5(7):428–439

Piburn S (1990) The Dalai Lama: A policy of kindness – An anthology of writings by and about the Dalai Lama, 2nd edn. Snow Lion Publications, Ithaca NY, pp. 16

Post SG (2007) Altruism and health: Perspectives from empirical research. Oxford University Press, Oxford UK

Radin D (2006) Entangled minds: Extrasensory experiences in a quantum reality. Paraview Pocket Books, New York NY

Radin DI, Stone J, Levine E, Eskandarnejad S, Schlitz M, Kozak L, Mandel D, Hayssen G (2008) Compassionate intention as a therapeutic intervention by partners of cancer patients: Effects of distant intention on the patients' autonomic nervous system. Explore: The Journal of Science and Healing 4(4):235–243

Schiltz M, Braud W (1997) Distant intentionality and healing: Assessing the evidence. Alternative Therapies in Health and Medicine 3(6):62–73

Stepanek MJT (2002) Heartsongs. Hachette Books, New York NY

Stepanek MJT, Carter J (2008) Just peace: A message of hope. Andrews McMeel Publishing, Kansas City MO

Yousafzai M (2015) I am Malala: The girl who stood up for education and was shot by the Taliban. Little, Brown and Company, New York NY

Chapter 15 – BREATHE in Action

Covey SR (1989) The seven habits of highly effective people: Powerful lessons in personal change. Free Press, New York NY

O'Donohue J (2008) To bless the space between us: A book of blessings. Doubleday, New York NY

Suggested Reading

Chapter 1 – Why Relationships Matter

Bolger N, Amarel D (2007) Effects of social support visibility on adjustment to stress: experimental evidence. Journal of Personality & Social Psychology 92:458–75

Bowlby J (1988) A secure base: Parent–child attachment and healthy human development. Basic Books, New York NY

Cassidy J, Shaver PR (2010) Handbook of attachment: Theory, research and clinical applications, 2nd edn. The Guilford Press, New York NY

Cozolino L (2014) The neuroscience of human relationships: Attachment and the developing social brain, 2nd edn. WW Norton & Company, New York NY

Goleman D (2004) Destructive emotions: A scientific dialogue with the Dalai Lama, reprint edn. Bantam Books, New York NY

Goleman D (2005) Emotional intelligence: Why it can matter more than IQ. Bantam Books, New York NY

Goleman D (2007) Social intelligence: The new science of human relationships, reprint edn. Bantam Books, New York NY

Gottman JM, Silver N (1999) The seven principles for making marriage work: A practical guide from the country's foremost relationship expert. Three Rivers Press, New York NY

Mikulincer M, Shaver PR (2010) Attachment in adulthood: Structure, dynamics and change. The Guilford Press, New York NY

Siegel DJ (2015) The developing mind: How relationships and the brain interact to shape who we are, 2nd edn. The Guilford Press, New York NY

Thorsteinsson EB, James JE (1999) A meta-analysis of the effects of experimental manipulations of social support during laboratory stress. Psychological Health 14:869–86

Chapter 2 – Understanding Stress

Dvorsky G (2013) Are we in the midst of an anxiety epidemic? Daily Explainer Nov. 16

Rauch SL, Shin LM, Wright CL (2003) Neuroimaging studies of amygdala function in anxiety disorders. Annals of the New York Academy of Sciences 985:389–410

Roosendaal B, McEwen BS, Chattarji S (2009) Stress, memory, and the amygdala. Nature Reviews Neuroscience 10:423–433

Sapolsky RM (1998) Why zebras don't get ulcers: An updated guide to stress-related disease and coping, 2nd edn. WH Freeman, London UK

Shin LM, Liberzon I (2010) The neurocircuitry of fear, stress, and anxiety disorders. Neuropsychopharmacology Reviews 35:169–191

Chapter 3 – Why Manage Chronic Stress?

Bremner JD (2005) Does stress damage the brain? Understanding trauma-related disorders from a mind–body perspective. WW Norton & Company, New York NY

Conrad C (2011) The handbook of stress: Neuropsychological effects on the brain. Wiley-Blackwell, Hoboken NJ

Porges SW (2011) Polyvagal theory. The neurophysiological foundations of emotions, attachment, communication, and self-regulation. WW Norton & Company, New York NY

Seery MD (2013) The biopsychological model of challenge and threat: using the heart to measure the mind. Social and Personality Compass 7(9):637–653

Taliaz D, Loya A, Gersner R, Haramati S, Chen A, Zangen A (2011) Resilience to chronic stress is mediated by hippocampal brain-derived neurotrophic factor. Journal of Neuroscience 31(12):4475–4483

Chapter 4 – The Stories We Tell: Why Mindset Matters

Dweck C (2007) Mindset: The new psychology of success. Ballantine Books, New York NY

Hayes SC, Barnes-Holmes D, Roche B (2001) Relational frame theory: A post-Skinnerian account of human language and cognition. Kluwer Academic/Plenum, New York NY, pp. 3–20

Ornstein PA (1995) Children's long-term retention of salient personal experiences. Journal of Traumatic Stress 8:581–606

Pennebaker JW, Smyth JM (2016) Opening up by writing it down: How expressive writing improves health and eases emotional pain, 3rd edn. The Guilford Press, New York NY

Siegel DJ (2010) Mindsight: The new science of personal transformation. Bantam Books, New York NY

Tucker DM, Lu P (2012) Cognition and neural development. Oxford University Press, Oxford UK

Turkle S (2011) Alone together: Why we expect more from technology and less from each other. Basic Books, New York NY

Chapter 5 – Mindfulness and the Mind

Begley S (2007) Train your mind, change your brain: How science reveals our extraordinary potential to transform ourselves. Ballantine Books, New York NY

Farias M, Wilkolm C (2015) The Buddha pill: Can meditation change you? Watkins Publishing, London UK

Feuerstein G (2001) The yoga tradition: Its history, literature, philosophy, and practice, 3rd edn. Hohm Press, Chino Valley AZ

Gelles D (2015) Mindful work: how meditation is changing business from the inside out. Houghton Mifflin Harcourt, New York NY

Hanley AW, Abell N, Osborn DS, Roehrig AD, Canto AI (2014) Mind the gaps: Are conclusions about mindfulness entirely conclusive? Journal of Counseling & Development 94:103–113

Heuman L (2014) Don't believe the hype: Neuroscientist Catherine Kerr is concerned about how mindfulness meditation research is being portrayed in the media. Tricycle [Online] Available at: http://tricycle.org/trikedaily/dont-believe-hype/

Iyengar BKS (1995) Light on yoga: yoga dipika. Schocken, New York NY

Kabat-Zinn J (1990) Full catastrophe living: Using the wisdom of your body and mind to face stress, pain, and illness. Delacorte, New York NY

Kabat-Zinn J (2003) Mindfulness-based interventions in context: past, present, and future. Clinical Psychology Science and Practice 10:144–155

Karatsoreos IN, McEwen BS (2013) Annual research review: The neurobiology and physiology of resilience and adaptation across the life course. The Journal of Child Psychology and Psychiatry 54(4):337–347

Marturano J (2015) Finding the space to lead. A practical guide to mindful leadership. Bloomsbury Press

National Center for Complementary & Integrative Health 2015 Report, DHHS. Meditation: what you need to know. National Center for Complementary and Integrative Health (NCCIH), Bethesda MD

Purser R, Loy D (2013) Beyond McMindfulness. The Huffington Post [Online] Available at: http://www.huffingtonpost.com/ron-purser/beyond-mcmindfulness_b_3519289.html

Shapiro SL, Carlson LE (2009) The art and science of mindfulness: Integrating mindfulness into psychology and the helping professions. American Psychological Association, Washington DC

Sykes Wylie M (2015) How the mindfulness movement went mainstream – and the backlash that came with it. Psychotherapy Networker, Alternet [Online] Available at: http://www.alternet.org/personal-health/how-mindfulness-movement-went-mainstream-and-backlash-came-it

Walsh W, Shapiro SL (2006) The meeting of meditative disciplines and Western psychology. American Psychologist 61(3):227–239

Chapter 6 – Personal Responsibility and Social Change

Poulin MJ, Brown SL, Dillard AJ, Smith DM (2013) Giving to others and the association between stress and mortality. American Journal of Public Health 103:1649–55

Powell JA (2015) Racing to justice: Transforming our conceptions of self and other to build an inclusive society. Indiana University Press, Bloomington IN

Senge P (2006) The fifth discipline: The art & practice of the learning organization, revised edn. Doubleday, New York NY

Chapter 7 – The BREATHE Model

Clarke T, Black LI, Stussman BJ, Barnes PM, Nahin RL (2015) Trends in the use of complementary health approaches among adults: United States, 2002–2012. National Health Statistics Reports 79

Rickard KB, Dunn DJ, Brouch VM (2015) Breathing techniques associated with improved health outcomes. Virginia Henderson Global Nursing e-Repository [Online] Available at: http://www.nursinglibrary.org/vhl/handle/10755/558648

Chapter 8 – Breath Awareness and Chapter 9 – Regulating the Autonomic Nervous System Through Intentional Breathing

Brown RP, Gerbarg PL (2012) The healing power of the breath: Simple techniques to reduce stress and anxiety, enhance concentration, and balance your emotions. Shambhala Publications Inc., Boston MA

Elliott S, Edmonson D (2006) The new science of the breath: coherent breathing for autonomic nervous system balance, health, and well-being. Coherence Press, Allen TX

Fried R (1999) Breathe well, be well: A program to relieve stress, anxiety, asthma, hypertension, migraine, and other disorders for better health. John Wiley & Sons, Inc., New York NY

Iyengar BKS (1985) Light on pranayama: The yogic art of breathing. The Crossroad Publishing Company, New York NY

Jerath R, Edry JW, Barnes VA, Jerath V (2006) Physiology of long pranayamic breathing: neural respiratory elements may provide a mechanism that explains how slow deep breathing shifts the autonomic nervous system. Medical Hypotheses 67(3):566–571

Ley R (1999) The modification of breathing behavior. Pavlovian and operant control in emotion and cognition. Behavior Modification 23:441–479

Rickard KB, Dunn DJ, Brouch VM (2015) Breathing techniques associated with improved health outcomes. Virginia Henderson Global Nursing e-Repository [Online] Available at: http://www.nursinglibrary.org/vhl/handle/10755/558648

Sovik R (2000) The science of breathing – The yogic view. Progress in Brain Research 122:491–505

van der Kolk B (2015) The body keeps the score: Brain, mind, and body in the healing of trauma. Viking, New York NY

Chapter 10 – Experiencing Emotion

Bolte Taylor J (2009) My stroke of insight: A brain scientist's personal journey. Plume, New York NY

Damasio A (1999) The feeling of what happens: Body and emotion in the making of consciousness. Harcourt, New York NY

Goleman D (2005) Emotional intelligence: Why it can matter more than IQ, 10th anniversary edn. Bantam Books, New York NY

McCraty R, Atkinson M (2003) Psychophysiological coherence, Publication 03-016. HeartMath Research Center, Institute of HeartMath, Boulder Creek CA

Mate G (2011) When the body says no: Exploring the stress–disease connection. Wiley, New York NY

Pollatos O, Gramann K, Schandry R (2007) Neural systems connecting interoceptive awareness and feelings. Human Brain Mapping 28(1):9–18

Radin DI, Schmitz MJ (2005) Gut feelings, intuition, and emotions: An exploratory study. The Journal of Alternative and Complementary Medicine 11(1):85–91

Schultz A, Vogele C (2015) Interception and stress. Frontiers in Psychology 6:993

Sternberg EM (2001) The balance within: The science connecting health and emotions. WH Freeman, London UK

Chapter 11 – Appraising and Adjusting Your Mindset

Dweck C (2007) Mindset: The new psychology of success. Ballantine Books, New York NY

Folkman S, Hammond KR (1999) Judgments under stress. Oxford University Press, Oxford UK

Singer MA (2007) The untethered soul. New Harbinger Publications Inc., Oakland CA

Weiner B (1995) Judgments of responsibility: A foundation for a theory of social conduct. The Guilford Press, New York NY

Chapter 12 – Taking a Purposeful Pause

Haslach C, Schaufelt WB, Leiter MP (2001) Job burnout. Annual Review of Psychology 52:397–422

Kabat-Zinn J (1994) Wherever you go, there you are. Hyperion, New York NY

Krystal AD (2012) Psychiatric disorders and sleep. Neurology Clinics 30(4):1389–1413

Chapter 13 – Humor: Life as Practice

Lefcourt HM, Martin RA (1986) Humor and life stress: antidote to adversity. Springer-Verlag, New York NY

Martin RA (2002) Is laughter the best medicine? Humor, laughter, and physical health. Current Directions in Psychological Science 11(6):216–220

Chapter 14 – Engaging Others Mindfully

Hatfield E, Cacioppo JT (1994) Emotional contagion: Studies in emotion and social interaction. Cambridge University Press, Cambridge UK

Iacoboni M (2009) Mirroring people: The science of empathy and how we connect with others. Picador, London UK

Inagaki TK, Bryne Haltom KE, Suzuki S, Jevtic I, Hornstein E, Bower JE, Eisenberger NI (2016) The neurobiology of giving versus receiving support. Psychosomatic Medicine 78(4):443–53

McTaggart L (2012) The bond: How to fix your falling-down world. Free Press, New York NY

Piburn S (1990) The Dalai Lama: A policy of kindness – An anthology of writings by and about the Dalai Lama, 2nd edn. Snow Lion Publications, Ithaca NY, pp. 16

Post SG (2007) Altruism and health: Perspectives from empirical research. Oxford University Press, Oxford UK

Radin D (2006) Entangled minds: Extrasensory experiences in a quantum reality. Paraview Pocket Books, New York NY

Stepanek MJT (2002) Heartsongs. Hachette Books, New York NY

Stepanek MJT, Carter J (2008) Just peace: A message of hope. Andrews McMeel Publishing, Kansas City MO

Yousafzai M (2015) I am Malala: The girl who stood up for education and was shot by the Taliban. Little, Brown and Company, New York NY

Chapter 15 – BREATHE in Action

Covey SR (1989) The seven habits of highly effective people: Powerful lessons in personal change. Free Press, New York NY

Index

Note: Page number followed by f and/or t indicates figure and table respectively.

Author Biography

B Grace Bullock, PhD, E-RYT 500 is a research scientist, psychologist, organizational innovator, author, educator, science journalist, and yoga and mindfulness expert. She received her PhD in Clinical Psychology from the University of Oregon, and BA Highest Honors, Summa Cum Laude in psychology, from the University of California at Los Angeles. Dr. Bullock served as Senior Scientist for the Ethics, Education and Human Development Initiative at the *Mind and Life Institute,* and Intervention Scientist at the *Institute of Neuroscience*, and the *Child and Family Center* at the *University of Oregon*. She is Founding Director of the *International Science & Education Alliance*, an organization devoted to research, program evaluation, strategic planning and capacity building to promote inclusion, diversity, and effective leadership and decision-making. She is Contributing Editor for Research at YogaU Online, and the former Editor-in-Chief of the *International Journal of Yoga Therapy*. You can learn more about her at www.bgrace-bullock.com

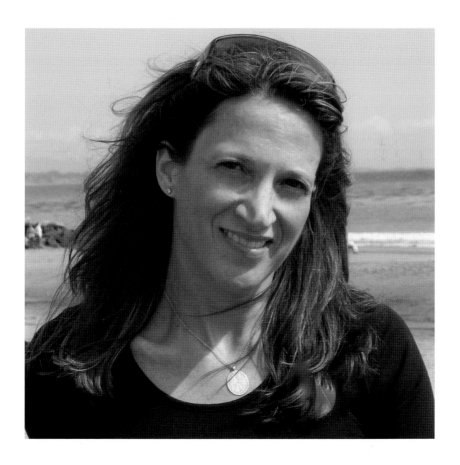